This book demonstrates one practical application of an emerging truth in the healing arts—that creating a positively energized home environment is an important aspect in recovery from any disorder, including brain trauma.

—Nikki Marie Welch, M.D., M.D.(H), Sedona, Arizona

This book is a page-turner. The author's humor and vivid writing drew me in immediately. I had to keep reading until I found out how these women, using their life experiences, made the impossible real.

—Suzanne Zuercher, clinical psychologist
and author of two books: *Enneagram Spirituality* and *Enneagram*

*Brain, Heal Thyself* is a compelling tale of resiliency and grace. Siles relates her experiences with honesty and humor, offering substantive insights to professionals, caregivers, and stroke victims themselves. Eve's ongoing recovery, which I've been privileged to witness, is testimony to the power and dignity of the human spirit. An inspiring, encouraging work.

—Thea Jarvis, Eve's college roommate and
author of *The Gift of Grandparenting*

*Brain, Heal Thyself* is a well-written, engaging story of devotion, tenacity and a miraculous recovery from devastating trauma.

—Thomas W. Phelan, Ph.D., author of
*1-2-3 Magic: Effective Discipline for Children 2–12*

# BRAIN, HEAL THYSELF

## A Caregiver's New Approach to Recovery from Stroke, Aneurysm, and Traumatic Brain Injuries

## MADONNA SILES

Commentary by Lawrence J. Beuret, M.D.

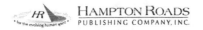

HAMPTON ROADS
PUBLISHING COMPANY, INC.

Cover design by Steve Amarillo
Cover art © Jupitermedia Corporation. All rights reserved.

Hampton Roads Publishing Company, Inc.
1125 Stoney Ridge Road
Charlottesville, VA 22902

434-296-2772
fax: 434-296-5096
e-mail: hrpc@hrpub.com
www.hrpub.com

If you are unable to order this book from your local
bookseller, you may order directly from the publisher.
Call 1-800-766-8009, toll-free.
Library of Congress Cataloging-in-Publication Data

Siles, Madonna.

Brain, heal thyself : a caregiver's new approach to recovery from stroke,
aneurysm, and traumatic brain injuries / Madonna Siles.
    p. cm.
Summary: "Part memoir, part recovery manual, Brain, Heal Thyself is a guidebook
for unexpected caregivers. Siles recounts moment-by-moment the journey of her
friend Eve's near-fatal aneurysm to ER to rehab center to at-home care and, finally, to
recovery. Includes visualizations and subliminal methods for invoking the power of
emotions and the subconscious mind in the healing process"--Provided by publisher.
    Includes bibliographical references and index.
    ISBN 1-57174-476-2 (5 1/2 x 8 1/2 tp : alk. paper)
    1. Cerebrovascular disease--Patients--Rehabilitation. 2. Cerebrovascular
disease--Patients--Biography. 3. Aneurysms--Patients--Rehabilitation. 4.
Aneurysms--Patients--Biography. 5. Brain--Wounds and injuries--Alternative
treatment. 6. Caregivers. I. Title.
    RC388.5.S49 2006
    362.196'810092--dc22
                                    2005037766

ISBN 1-57174-476-2
10 9 8 7 6 5 4 3
Printed on acid-free paper in Canada

*To my parents, Mary and Steve,*
*who gave me the good life . . .*
*and to my A.A. friends and sponsors*
*who taught me how to live it*

# Contents

## Part Two: Riding the Roller Coaster to Recovery

# Acknowledgments

Without the 12-Step program of Alcoholics Anonymous, Eve and I would never have met. Now, how much fun would that have been? Thanks, Eve, for sharing the past 12 years with me as we "trudge the road of happy destiny."

In addition, I have relied on the feedback of friends and experts while writing this book. Thank you, Valerie Samuelson and Peggy Savides, R.N., for your invaluable input at every stage of this book. Special thanks to Kevin Beuret, who edited the final manuscript.

My gratitude extends to my commentators and cheerleaders, including: Fran Holdren, Jennifer Berns, Gloria Muczynski, Chrissy Shults, Jean Handel-Bailey, Fran Corn, Karen Piwowarski, Patricia Fanella-DeVito, Gina Ward, Thea Jarvis, Cathy Causby, Paul Savides, Neil O'Shea, Deborah Fleck, Tania Seymour, Sara Sgarlat, Mark Knoblauch, Carol Morgan, Ph.D., and Sue Powers, R.N.

I am also forever grateful for the support of my friends Merle, the late (great) Roger Ketelsen, and Patricia Moeller, who lost her battle with cancer a year ago. I miss Roger and Pat very much. There are many others who helped Eve and me on the road to recovery in many different ways. They include: Yolanda, Ginny, Arlene and Jim Smith, Penny and Ron Latko, Alex and Lynn, Carlie Koss, Chuck Kaleta, Norm and Doris, Jim Berns, Eileen, G. J., Greg, Dan Rubino, Carolyn Halenza, Laura, Marion, Mary, Auntie Simone, Tony Costanza, Bruce Shivley, Alice Grippe, Carol Stevenson, Peg, Laurie, Diana, Kathy White, and Nikki Welch, M.D. We thank you.

We are indebted to the health professionals who went beyond their professional calling to help Eve and to support me.

Special thanks to Max Ots, M.D.; Tracy Bielinski, R.N.; Mary Vietzke, R.N.; Sharon Prosser, B.S.W.; Julie Feld, M.S.W.; Patti Seeman, C.O.T.A.; Leo Grieben, M.D.; Karen Butler, M.D.; and Bonnie Davis. Many others were there with kind acts or encouraging words when we needed them. If I had known I was going to write a book, I would have recorded all their names. You know who you are. We thank you, one and all. May God bless you.

# Foreword

In 1987, my eight-year-old daughter experienced a serious brain injury when she was hit by a car. In 1995, the teenaged son of friends sustained a head injury when he was a backseat passenger in a car that went off the road and rolled several times. Most recently, another family's son, a 21-year-old soldier in the U.S. Army in Iraq, incurred serious brain damage when a roadside bomb blew up his vehicle.

A litany of tragedies, yes, and each was followed by a lengthy and expensive hospitalization. When these patients finally went home, another trauma occurred, but this time it did not happen to the patients. It happened to the caregivers. They were suddenly thrust into the role of caregivers to a brain-injured person. Totally unprepared and armed only with love and an urgent desire to "bring them back," they took over where hospital rehabilitation left off.

When my daughter came home from the hospital, many people commented that our family was lucky because I was a registered nurse. They implied that my professional training had equipped me with the knowledge and skills to manage recovery at home. Nothing could have been further from the truth!

The fact is, nobody is really prepared to care for someone with a brain injury or stroke. It would have been great to have a set of instructions or a rehabilitation formula to follow, but instead almost everything we were told or read contained the qualifier: "Every brain injury is different."

Thankfully, in *Brain, Heal Thyself*, Ms. Siles invites us to look for the similarities between her case and ours. She proceeds to apply the universal rules of nonverbal, subconscious communication to her brain-recovery situation and asks us to do the same. Then she surprises us by employing advertising strategies as rehabilitation motivational tools and 12-Step program concepts to facilitate the two-way communication process. It certainly appears that these positive methods work much better than the cajoling, controlling, bribing, and browbeating we were often reduced to when we got frustrated.

In the years that our daughter was recovering, there were few support services available for brain injuries, and even fewer for the caregivers. Then, as now, we searched for answers in self-help materials. At last we have found what we were looking for—creative rehabilitation ideas, inspiration to develop our own new methods, and recovery hope without unrealistic expectations—in my friend's book, *Brain, Heal Thyself*.

—Peggy Savides, R.N.

# Preface

In the following pages, I have relived the experience of my friend Eve's near-fatal brain aneurysm/stroke, her rehabilitation and recovery, and my attempts to help as her primary, nonprofessional caregiver.

I was—am—the original clueless caregiver. As you read, you will notice that this memoir is devoid of professional medical terms. That's because, in most cases, I can't spell them. Likewise, very few explanations are attributed to medical professionals. That's because there weren't many. Though Eve's medical records are in my possession, I can't make heads or tails of the indecipherable notes made by doctors, nurses, and laboratory technicians. This is a sad statement coming from a college graduate with a degree in communications.

My inability to grasp the gravity of Eve's condition during her first days in the hospital caused me to make some decisions that could have had dire consequences for both of us. Perhaps if I had been more assertive—if I had asked more questions about Eve's chances for survival versus quality of life—I could have avoided a lot of emotional turmoil. I sincerely hope you never have to endure that level of fear and emotional pain.

That's why I am sharing this story with you. The concerned medical and rehabilitation professionals may challenge my interpretation of the events, their prognoses, and their treatment methods. I have never doubted that these professionals were trying to do their best for Eve under the circumstances, but this is the way I remember the ordeal.

I don't believe I would have survived physically, mentally, or emotionally without practicing the principles of the 12-Step program. So, in that spirit, I will proceed to share my experience, strength, and hope with you. As the program suggests: You may take what you need . . . and leave the rest.

# Introduction

On October 11, 2001, an otherwise ordinary day, an exploding brain aneurysm, a cerebral hemorrhage, catapulted my friend Eve to the waiting room outside heaven's gates. However, they didn't have room for her that day. This was fortunate, or unfortunate, as you will read later on. Over the next few weeks, I, the caregiver, descended into the hellish limbo of "let's wait and see." While the medical professionals were predicting a probable "vegetable" outcome for Eve, her brain was beginning to recover . . . and it seemed nobody was noticing except me.

What I learned from this experience was that the brain aneurysm happened to both of us, devastating our lives in different ways. I began to recover first, which was good since I was the caregiver.

This is an upside-down book, filled with paradoxes aplenty. Caregiving was a role I never wanted and did everything under the sun to avoid . . . except run away. In the process of sticking around, I was transformed from a confused, frightened caregiver to a brain trauma rehabilitator. Since nobody could tell me how to perform in my new role, I "invented" my own strategy for creating a recovery environment and therapy routine that encouraged my friend's brain to heal itself.

Early on, I realized that, in today's medical/insurance/social services environment, there is no financial motivation and therefore no "system" in place for long-term professional rehabilitation of stroke or TBI (traumatic brain injury) survivors. After the basic hospital fix-up, a month-long in-hospital therapy program, and ten or so outpatient sessions, the "system" bows out. Depending on the patient's ability to function at home, most caregivers are faced with the choice between a nursing home and at-home care. Without extraordinary insurance coverage or Medicaid, the choice of the nursing home stay is an unaffordable luxury for most average-income families, so the whole puzzling situation comes home to roost. But at least at home the survivor won't be ignored and will constantly receive the individualized attention the brain requires.

Even though hospice plans, visiting nurse organizations, and private caregiving businesses are springing up all over, they have little to offer the brain trauma survivor in terms of rehabilitation. In the end, the caregiver must rely on his/her own resources and a few photocopied therapy routines, compliments of the rehabilitation center.

One would think that in this era of instant Internet information, online support organizations, and self-help books, there would be resources galore for this debilitating condition that plagues hundreds of thousands of Americans!

For those of you who have "been there, done that," you already know that maddening qualifier that's on almost every website or in each home therapy book: "Every stroke is different." That means they can tell us how to strengthen a weakened limb or how to play memory games—but don't push them to answer our weird questions.

Someday, try surfing the Internet for a "cure" for a condition I call "no body-function feedback." That's when the stroke patient has no awareness of when they are freezing and shivering, boiling and sweating, when their nose is running (or how to blow it), when to cough, the need to pee (or even realize it's too late), inappropriately laughing, burping, belching, or humming to themselves for hours on end. I suppose the good news is that it's not a life-threatening condition, except, of course, for the caregiver who can't take it anymore.

But there are many other such caregiver questions that are life or health threatening that also can't be answered in general. How do you *know* when it's really safe to teach someone to shower by herself when she still loses her balance 30 percent of the time? How do you teach someone to cook who is seemingly capable of all the stages except remembering to turn off the stove? And here's one guaranteed to give a caregiver sleepless nights: When is it safe to let the stroke patient drive a car to the grocery store—alone? These are the questions that keep the caregiver stuck in the enabling phase rather than rising to rehabilitator status.

You might be operating under the illusion that health professionals with a string of initials after their names have the correct answers to these questions. On occasion, I myself have bought into that illusion. But in reality, you, the home caregiver, are the best qualified to make these decisions. Scary, huh?

Paradoxically speaking, if I had been surrounded by friends with medical credentials before I started, I would have given up. Even the most caring professionals told me that I could not greatly influence Eve's recovery. No doubt, these friends would have convinced me to go back to work, leaving Eve to flounder through the day under the watchful eye of a paid caregiver/babysitter. She would have somehow survived. But this book would never have been written because I'd have nothing to say. Instead, not only did I write it, but Eve typed and proofread every page.

In the end, I hope that my book will give you the same level of confidence in your decision-making capabilities for your loved one's rehabilitation that the health professionals spent years in acquiring. As you read, you'll see how I transformed myself into a rehabilitator through a process called "ego-deflation" (a term you will not find in most doctors' vocabularies). I loosely define it as "life happens and I must accept it and change." Simple to understand, but not so easy to do. It takes willingness. But by coming to grips with my shortcomings as a caregiver, and acknowledging the chaos created by our brain trauma situation, I was paradoxically given the power to handle the caregiving/rehabilitation decision-making process with confidence. If it sounds familiar, then you'll know I "borrowed" the concept from the 12-Step program.

Perhaps you're wondering who could possibly have "ego" problems in the midst of a brain trauma crisis. Not you, of course, but maybe you can identify with some of my typical ego reactions during a crisis. My favorite is "Poor me, no one understands my pain," or "Please help me, I can't do this." Then we have "I'll show you, you can't tell me what to do," or "How can you do this to us?" Helpless, whiney, depressed, frustrated, fearful, and indignant—I was all this and more. The feelings are valid, but totally unproductive in a caregiving/rehabilitation situation. More than any other time in my life, I had to learn to acknowledge my character defects, get over them quickly, and then do a constructive action in the right direction.

I will also discuss another daunting challenge facing most brain trauma caregivers: the need to forsake control over the outcome of their efforts, and to learn to accept their powerlessness over progress in the recovery process.

The injured brain will recover at its own rate, with very little thanks to the well-meaning, beleaguered caregiver's pleas, plans, efforts, or prayers. In other words, "No matter how one beats at the portals of night, daylight will come at the appointed hour."

By surrendering to my powerlessness in the rehabilitation situation (another 12-Step program concept), I was paradoxically empowered to try any rehabilitation technique that came to mind.

As you will see, the rehabilitation strategy I devised for Eve combined creative visualizations, advertising techniques, and the 12-Step program teaching method (aka sponsorship). All are aimed at teaching or motivating behavior changes by appealing to the often elusive and misunderstood, but amazingly powerful, subconscious mind. Though how the subconscious operates remains mostly a mystery, all three of these methods are generally acknowledged as capable of affecting a change in the subconscious domain.

As I describe my simple exercises with Eve, you'll realize you don't have to be a rocket scientist to harness the powers of the subconscious and make them work for you in the brain trauma rehabilitation situation.

In fact, the most challenging aspect may be changing yourself into a relatively relaxed and receptive caregiver. Taking care of yourself physically/mentally/emotionally is an absolute requirement for the subconscious healing process to work both ways. And this may be the major paradox in this book: By caring for himself or herself, the caregiver is able to create the hopeful environment where miracles can happen, where the injured brain, as if by magic, can heal itself.

# PART ONE

# ALL ABOARD THE MERRY-GO-ROUND OF MEDICAL CARE

# 1

# The Brain Bomb Explodes

It is another astounding Indian summer afternoon in Door County, the northeast Wisconsin peninsula that juts into the sky-blue waters of Green Bay and Lake Michigan. The misty atmosphere virtually vibrates with the jewel tones of nature—garnet, sapphire, topaz, and ruby—all set in shimmering gold. No wonder Door County is the Midwest's artists' Mecca. The patio door of my harbor-side home is wide open to an unusually balmy breeze off Lake Michigan. I've been lured to my easel by the siren call of seagulls, lapping waves, and chirping backyard birds. Puffs of clouds are racing seagulls across the cobalt sky. Truly, this is paradise. Nothing can ruin my ecstatic mood as I paint the spectacular landscape I can see from my studio.

Earlier in the partly cloudy day, I had been moping around, still trying to recover from a weeklong bout with bronchitis. My housemate and best friend, Eve, had not too subtly suggested I get some fresh air by mowing the lawn before she gave the yard a final trim for the season.

Despite my initial reluctance, mowing turned out to be no chore at all. It was invigorating. As the sun claimed more and more of the sky, the temperature responded accordingly, eventually creating a perfect fall day. I even thanked Eve for getting me moving again.

Now I feel good enough to return to my painting, while Eve zips around the yard with her weed whip. As the birch shadows lengthen in the late afternoon sun, I am totally lost in the mesmerizing process of creativity. Certainly, it takes me several minutes before I realize that the weed whip is silent, replaced by anguished cries of distress mixed with the background noise of nature.

"Help me! Help me!" The words finally register in my mind.

Oh, Lord, I wonder if Eve has chopped off a hand or foot. Dropping the paintbrush, I race out of my art studio into the dining room.

I hear the cry again, but I don't know where it's coming from. Sound plays tricks in a lakefront house. I run out on the deck. She's not in the yard. Back inside, I fly through the kitchen to the front door. Nope, not there. Maybe the laundry room? Bathroom? Where is she? I hurry into the living room and peer down the dark hallway to our side door. There she is! Eve crawls out of the hallway shadows and collapses at my feet, moaning, "Help me."

At first, I'm frozen, then panicked. "What happened?" I shriek. "Did you cut off a foot?" Quickly checking, I'm relieved. No blood. Her legs and hands are intact. Thank God, I don't have to retrieve a body part from a bush.

Eve is crawling again to the middle of the living room. Now she's rolling around on the rug, legs thrashing, clutching her head in her hands. She's berserk with pain.

"What's the matter? Please tell me." I'm begging for an answer.

"Don't know. Felt like I was shot between my eyes. Fell to my knees . . . passing out . . . crawled in . . . God, the pain!" The words come tumbling out in one breathless rush.

I lean over and check her head. Maybe a stone hit her? Maybe a wayward bullet? It's deer hunting season, isn't it? Nope, no holes. Suddenly, she's quiet. I'm grateful for the silence. Then I notice that her eyes are rolling back. It appears she's losing consciousness.

# The Brain Bomb Explodes

"Eve, are you fainting?"

"Going to be sick."

"No, wait," I squeak, "not on the living room rug." Like a raving lunatic, I run into the kitchen and fling open the cabinets, looking for a plastic bowl. An old one. What's the matter with me? Just go help her, stupid. Then a thought occurs. Hey, wait a second. This is probably just a migraine. Eve gets one every other month. Sometimes she vomits. Yep, that's what it is, a dumb headache.

I hurry to the living room and thrust the old bowl at her face in the nick of time. I close my eyes until she's finished gagging. Nervously, I check in the bowl. Uh-oh. It doesn't look like lunch, nor does it look normal. "Please," I beseech her, "tell me, do you think this is a migraine?"

No answer. She's losing consciousness again. She's never done that before.

I jump up and run to the phone. "Eve, is this migraine or should I call 9-1-1?" I wave the receiver in the air threateningly. Precious moments pass.

"Call," she says weakly.

As Eve passes out, I punch the buttons.

"Emergency operator."

"I'm not sure. I think we need help. An ambulance. My room-mate hurt her head somehow. She's losing consciousness. I don't know if it's a migraine." I vaguely hope the operator will shed some light on my dilemma. "I think she's unconscious now."

"Where are you?" the calming voice asks.

"In Baileys Harbor." I recite the street directions. It feels like I'm talking in slow motion. "Yes, the driveway is on the right coming from Sturgeon Bay."

This is going to take forever, I think. Sturgeon Bay is 40 minutes away. But no sooner do I hang up than there is a pounding at the backdoor. Who needs visitors now?

I run to see who's there. It's the owner of a restaurant down the street. She's holding a duffel bag. Really, I don't have time to chat now.

"I just got the emergency call," she says breathlessly. "I'm a

5

medical first responder. I know CPR. What's wrong? Is it your roommate?"

"Oh, yes, she's in the living room. Thank you. Please hurry." As I open the door, I see two more first responders running up the driveway. I wave them inside and direct them to the living room. Amazing. Where are these people coming from?

"Does Eve have a heart attack history?" a responder asks. "How about stroke?"

"No," I answer. "No!"

Now the three first responders are kneeling next to Eve. "Well, it might be a migraine," one says. "We need some ice."

I run to the refrigerator. Another knock at the door. Another first responder.

"Get some blankets," someone shouts. "She might be in shock."

I know I am in shock. I'm racing around like the proverbial headless chicken. I retrieve the ice from the refrigerator and run to the linen closet to find a blanket. Where are the damn blankets? Oh yeah, way up on the top shelf. I pull one and they all come tumbling down.

I hear the distant wail of a siren. Wow, that ambulance got here fast. Soon there's another knock at the door. "Paramedics," they shout in unison.

Armed with oxygen and a stretcher, they quickly take over. I'm crowded out of the living room trauma scene. Standing in the doorway, I feel so helpless as they call out more of the same questions. They're all shouting at Eve to stay awake. I overhear one of them talking to the hospital on his cell phone. "Might be a migraine," one paramedic says. "I don't think so," counters the other.

In the blink of an eye, they've strapped petite Eve onto the stretcher. The first responders rise in unison as they watch the medics cart Eve down the hallway and out the door. The first responders parade out behind them. As if it's an afterthought, one paramedic runs back into the house to talk to me.

"We're transporting Eve to the Door County hospital in Sturgeon Bay. You'll have to drive yourself." She turns and heads back to the ambulance.

As quickly as they came, they're gone. Standing alone in the kitchen, I'm not sure what to do next. First, I better change from my grubby painting attire. My hands are filthy. What a sight. The spooked cats, Ozzie and Lola, are meowing loudly for their dinner. My head's throbbing; I'm not over the bronchitis yet. Wish I had taken a nap earlier. I feel intensely sleepy; it's my own peculiar reaction to panic. Not a very helpful defense mechanism at the moment.

Robotically, I proceed through the tasks at hand. I'm unsuccessful at calming the cats, but I manage to divert their attention by throwing food in their bowls. Next, I ransack Eve's desk drawers, searching for the medical power of attorney documents. I haven't a clue where they are. Eve is keeper of the business papers. Eventually, I find the old Illinois power of attorney (POA), a relic of our Chicago past. It'll have to do. Finally I lock up the house and head to the hospital.

All the way to Sturgeon Bay, I browbeat myself. Why, oh why, did I call an expensive ambulance instead of putting Eve to bed? This will probably cost us $500 that we can't afford. Of course, it must be a migraine headache. She has a history of them. Eve was obviously overacting and, as usual, I am overreacting.

I hate to admit I'm so squeamish. My nursing skills are limited to fixing a cup of tea or dispensing an aspirin. If the situation gets any messier than that, I recommend calling a doctor. This time, however, my immaturity is going to cost us big bucks. I'll bet the ambulance crew was snickering all the way to Sturgeon Bay, making fun of the ditzy lady who cried "wolf" when it was only a lamb.

I arrive at the hospital and haul my bruised ego into the emergency center. A receptionist directs me to Eve's room. She is sitting up in bed, looking a little dazed. No one else is in the room. I fear that Eve's going to reprimand me for sending her off in an ambulance.

"How's your head?" I ask.

"It really hurts."

"Do they think it's a migraine?"

"Not sure."

Just then, a doctor bursts through the door, followed by a nurse. Two unfamiliar paramedics are trailing behind.

"Who are you?" he asks me bluntly. I explain that I am Eve's roommate.

He frowns. "So you're not a blood relative?"

"No, but I have this power of attorney paper." He smiles. Obviously, I said the magic words. He grabs the paper, and nods as he peruses the document.

"Okay, here's the situation. We've performed a CT scan and detected blood on her brain. Our diagnosis is a subarachnoid hemorrhage. We don't have the facilities to treat a cerebral hemorrhage here, so we're transferring her to Green Bay. First, we need you to sign these papers." He nods to the nurse, as he exits to answer a ringing phone.

"I'll sign," Eve pipes up in a meek little voice.

The nurse bypasses me and hands Eve the clipboard. Looking over her shoulder, I see Eve scrawl something. It sure doesn't look like her signature. I feel sick now.

The nurse looks at the signature doubtfully. "Here, you better countersign," she says to me. "And you look a little green. Why don't you sit down for a minute?"

The doctor reappears. "We've just received confirmation that a neurosurgeon is standing by waiting for Eve's arrival at the hospital in Green Bay. We've already called a long-distance ambulance company to take her."

At this, the two paramedics step forward to shake my hand. "I'm Rose. I'll be driving the ambulance. We want you to leave right now for the hospital. We'll pass you on the highway with lights flashing and sirens going. Don't be alarmed, that's just the way we drive. You stick to the speed limit, understand? Stay calm."

"Can't I go with you? I don't know where the hospital is," I whine.

"No, you can't. Joe, here, is writing out directions for you. Now get going." She touches my cheek sympathetically.

"Here, honey. Don't worry. I'll be riding in back with your friend. I'll take good care of her, I promise," Joe says, as he gives my shoulder a reassuring pat.

I believe him.

# 2

# No Extraordinary Measures

As I drive down State Highway 57, the setting sun's last rays are lighting up the clouds gathering over Green Bay. It looks a little ominous out there. Amazingly, I'm not at all tempted to speed. In fact, I'm driving about five miles under the limit. Truth is: I don't want to go to Green Bay. I'm playing with the idea that if I run away, the problem will go away. That's what I want to do. Just keep driving past Green Bay, through the cornfields of Iowa, across the plains of Nebraska, all the way to the Colorado Rockies. Perhaps the Pacific Ocean. Anywhere but here. Actually, I have no idea what a cerebral hemorrhage is. Is it life threatening? Is this trip a precautionary measure? Heck, what's a little blood on the brain, anyway? Can't the doctor just go in there and sop it up with a sponge? My mind hops from one solution to another, searching for a comforting thought.

Green Bay, next exit. Despite my desire to run, I dutifully turn off the highway and continue down side streets to northeast Wisconsin's regional brain trauma center.

Turning into the hospital driveway, I notice a sign for valet parking. How about that? Don't know why I'm so surprised. Green Bay isn't exactly a small rural town. I drive up and lower the window to ask for directions to the emergency entrance.

The friendly faced valet says, "Evening, ma'am. I'll park your car. Walk through those double doors, go down the hall, and turn right."

Inside, the lobby is deserted. It's a sight I've never seen at 8 P.M. in a Chicagoland hospital. It looks like everyone, including the staff, has gone home for the night. My footsteps echo down the empty corridor. Rounding the corner, I run smack into Joe, the ambulance paramedic.

He grabs my shoulders. "I'm sorry, honey. But we had a serious problem on the way here. Eve suffered a grand mal seizure in the ambulance. She's in critical condition. Run, don't walk, to the fifth floor neuro-ICU."

My body freezes in place. I'm stupefied. What happened? I thought he said he would take care of her. My mind is totally blank. All I can do is stand there and stare at Joe in stunned disbelief.

"Come with me," he says kindly. "I'll take you upstairs." Then he turns me around and pushes me toward a bank of elevators.

The elevator ascends in slow motion. Finally, the doors open on the fifth floor. The scene before me is utter pandemonium. Four nurses are gathered around a crash cart, clapping their hands and shouting, "Wake up!" I cautiously approach. One nurse sees me and calls out, "Are you her friend?"

I look and nod dumbly.

"Here, see if you can wake her." There's urgency in her voice. She pushes me to the front, as the nurses part.

"Eve," I whisper hoarsely. "It's me. Wake up." Eve's eyes are tightly closed; her skin is sickly pale. No response.

Okay, I'll try again a little louder. "Please, wake up." No response. Time to get tough. In a voice that would wake the dead, I bellow, "Eve, wake up now!"

Eve's eyes fly open. "Huh, what?" she asks, then shuts her eyes again.

"Great! Okay. Let's go!" the nurse commands, as she grabs my sleeve. "You come, too."

The nurses move so quickly down the hall with the cart that I have to run to keep up with them. We all crowd into another elevator. Eve looks dead to me. A nurse informs me that we're on our way to radiology for pictures of Eve's brain. The elevator opens on a darkened reception area; a desk lamp is the only source of illumination.

"Where's the radiologist?" the panicked ICU nurse asks a girl sitting behind a desk.

"We've paged him. He's on the way." The girl rises from the desk and steps out of the shadows. She must be the radiology technician, but she looks so young.

The ICU nurse is impatient. "We've got to get this patient hooked up. Now! She's hanging on by a thread."

"We're setting up the equipment," the tech replies. She's backing up to the door, away from the threatening ICU nurse. "Go ahead. Take her in."

If I had any cookies to toss, I would've done so at that moment. Sheer panic pervades the atmosphere. The nurses bulldoze their way through a door with the cart and disappear into a harshly lit room. The door closes on them, but I can still feel the panic.

At that moment, an outside door opens and a handsome young guy in a jogging outfit runs in, waves hi to me, and continues on into the room. His Nikes look brand-new. In a flash, he's back.

"Hi, I'm Dr. Jenkins, the radiologist," he says with a movie-star smile. "I came as quickly as I could. While they're setting up, let's look at the scans from Sturgeon Bay and I'll explain what's happening to your friend."

He spreads pictures of Eve's skull on a light box. "Hmmm," he says. "It appears she's had a brain aneurysm. See? This area here is the blood on her brain." He makes a sweeping hand circle.

I have no idea what I'm looking at. Which area? Is it black or white or gray? Who cares? Whatever, it seems to me to be everywhere.

"Well, they should be ready for me now. The neurosurgeon upstairs needs our scans to decide whether to operate. He'll talk to you then. But, for now, why don't you sit in that waiting room down there?" He points down a dimly lit hallway. "We're hurrying, but it's still going to take some time. We'll come for you when we're done."

In the darkened waiting room, I manage to discern a lamp in the shadows and switch it on. I scan the room for a pay phone and then realize there's a phone right next to me on a magazine-covered table. Hope I have my calling card. I check my wallet. Here it is! But whom should I call? All of our close friends are five hours away in Chicago.

Since Eve and I devoted our first year in Baileys Harbor to rehabbing our 50-year-old house, we barely know our next-door neighbors, let alone anyone else in town or Door County.

But it's getting late; nearly 10 P.M. Must have lost some time in the black hole of panic. I'd better call somebody to calm me down. Maybe Cass.

Digging in my purse, I find Cass's crumpled business card. She's Eve's closest friend down in Naperville, Illinois, our old stomping grounds.

Cass and Eve had met about ten years ago in a golf league. At that time, Eve was a year into her young widowhood. Her husband had died of cancer complications at the age of 48. Cass had just lost her husband, 43, to a heart attack. She had said, "He was dead before he hit the ground." Anyway, their friendship had grown as together they coped with their tragic losses and sudden single status. When I met Eve, we became a threesome.

Luckily, her home phone number is on the card. "Please be home. Please be awake. Please pick up," I pray as the phone keeps ringing.

"Hello," a sleepy voice mumbles.

"Hi, Cass. It's Donna," my voice cracks. "Sorry. Did I wake you?"

"What's wrong?"

"Oh, God, Cass, Eve has had a brain aneurysm. At least, that's what they told me. She's unconscious. She had a seizure in the ambulance." Now I'm whimpering and shaking so hard I can barely hold the phone.

Cass takes an audible deep breath. "Okay. Calm down. Where are you? I'm coming up."

Relief washes over me. She cares! "No, don't come up tonight, Cass. It's a five-hour trip. The deer are out. It's too risky. Eve's unconscious anyway. What could you do?"

"Calm you down, for one thing."

"It's okay. I'll get it together. I feel calmer already, just talking to you."

"Where's Eve now?"

"In radiology. The surgeon needs a brain scan before he can decide what to do. That's all I know right now. I'll be meeting with him soon."

"All right, here's my plan. First, I'll call somebody from the office to cover for me tomorrow. Hmmm, I need somebody to watch the cat, too. But I can leave here at 6 A.M. Where should we meet?"

"I'll call you on your cell phone tomorrow and give you directions." Out of the corner of my eye, I see the young tech signaling me. "Gotta go, Cass. I think they want me upstairs."

"Calm down. I'll say a prayer. Good luck. Call me anytime if something happens."

"Thanks." I hang up quickly. Stomach's churning again. The calmness was short-lived. The tech guiding me to the elevator bank tells me Eve's already been taken upstairs.

Finally, the elevator arrives. Alone again, I begin the slow ascent to hell.

When the doors open, I'm greeted by a forty-ish man in a navy business suit. His blue eyes twinkle under slicked-back blond hair. His grand moustache highlights a warm smile. Holding out his hand, he introduces himself as Dr. Brum (not his real name), the neurosurgeon. I detect an accent. German?

He takes me into his office and motions toward a chair. I brace myself for the news.

"Are you a relative of Eve's?" he asks.

"No, I'm her friend, Donna Siles, her roommate. We moved here from Chicago. There's no one else around. But I have power of attorney."

He smiles. "Good. Well, your friend has had a very bad brain aneurysm. That means a weakened blood vessel has burst in her brain, spraying it with blood. Understand? Normally, I would wait 24 hours before operating. But I fear she will not make it through the night without surgery. I must operate immediately and clip the aneurysm to stop it from bleeding. Do you understand?"

"I think so," I lie. "Is the surgery dangerous?"

"No, the surgery is not that risky. It's the 48-hour recovery period that's critical. Does Eve have an advance directive?" he asks. "I need to know her wishes concerning life support."

Alarm bells start ringing in my head as I hand him the medical power of attorney document, including the advance directive. I've had this life support discussion before, when my parents were dying of cancer. In my mother's case, I learned that the question of life support is never simple or clear-cut.

"No life support," I say slowly, emphatically. "It's Eve's wish. It's my wish." Then I sit back in the chair, waiting for the inevitable "but."

He peruses the paper. "I see. No extraordinary measures." He looks up. "But following the surgery, we will need to put Eve on a breathing apparatus. Her brain will recover more quickly without the additional burden of breathing control. Do you understand? I need your consent. We've got to give her a chance, right? She's only 55. She's too young."

"Yes, I'll consent to that." My head is nodding yes, but my brain is screaming, "No! No! You'll regret it!"

"Good. Now, if everything goes well, I expect Eve will be in ICU for a week and in a regular hospital bed for another week, maybe two. Then she'll be admitted to our inpatient hospital rehabilitation program for a month."

"A month?" The words jump out of my mouth. "What kind of rehab takes a month?" Clearly, I do not comprehend the consequences of a cerebral hemorrhage.

The surgeon sighs. "Eve has already suffered extensive brain damage in the personality and communications sector of her brain. She will never be the same. She'll have difficulty communicating and processing information. She'll have memory loss. Her mood will be changed. She'll be subdued, probably depressed."

My mind rejects most of his words of doom. I can't—won't— believe it. Instead, I focus on visualizing a subdued Eve. The vision does not compute.

"But brain damage can be reversed, can't it?" I protest. "Eve's smart, a college grad. She reads all the time. She's outgoing. Can't the damage be reversed?" I'm pleading for a positive response.

"Possibly," he says hesitantly. "But only time will tell. Now I have to prepare to operate," he says, rising from the chair. "Are you staying in the ICU waiting room for the night or going home?"

"I don't know." I agonize with the decision to stay or go. I'm not feeling well; the bronchitis is coming back. "I think I better go home." I desperately want to wake up in my own bed and discover this is just a nightmare.

"Good idea. You don't look well. Listen, everything should be okay. I'll call you if something goes wrong. Otherwise, assume the surgery is a success. It could take four or five hours. Go get some sleep."

As he opens the door, we're greeted by a skinny guy with owl eyes and oversized glasses. He says, "Miss Siles? We need to talk. Follow me, please."

As we walk down the hall, he introduces himself as the pastoral care director. Maybe he wants to say a prayer for Eve? Okay with me, I could use some spiritual solace now.

The moment we're seated in his office, he gets right down to business. "I understand you're not a blood relative," he says accusingly, "and you have a power of attorney document. May I see it, please?"

My goodness, word travels quickly. I hand it over.

"While I read this, please fill out these admissions forms." He pushes a pile of papers toward me.

I race through the forms. Finished. He's still reading the POA very carefully, taking a long time. Perhaps if he cleaned his glasses, he could read it faster. I just want to go home.

"Who is this second person listed here?"

"Eve's cousin, Vivian, in Chicago."

"Oh, good, a blood relative. Why didn't she sign the power of attorney paper?"

"I don't know. I didn't notice she hadn't," I reply. Damn, I thought Eve handled that way back when.

"Well, we have to call her right now," he says, pushing the phone toward me.

"No, we don't," I retaliate. "It's nearly midnight. She and her husband are in bed. She never answers the phone after nine. Her answering machine will take the message."

"Fine. Then leave her a message to contact this office or you. We need the medical POA signed this weekend."

He wins. I leave a message for her to call me first thing in the morning. Then he makes another request. "You have to select a local funeral home now."

"A what?" I stutter. "Why?" Geez, maybe Eve died while I was meeting with the surgeon. I haven't actually seen her for several hours. I start shaking again. "Is Eve dead?"

"No, she's in surgery," he calmly replies. "But she arrived in critical condition. In the event she dies, where do you want us to send her body? A funeral home in Door County?" He looks down at the checklist in front of him. How very efficient.

"I haven't had a chance to think about it," I reply, not as sarcastically as I might on a good day. "I guess I'd ship her to Chicago. That's where her friends are. Her parents owned a funeral home. They sold it to, um, Blake-Lamb. They have so many locations; I'm not sure which one I'd choose. Probably one near Naperville. Eve lived there for 20 years and . . ." I stop talking, realizing I'm babbling.

"Well, we need you to pick a local Green Bay funeral home. That's where she'd go first; then they ship the body to Chicago." He hands me the yellow pages. "Pick one."

Oh, for heavens' sakes. This is insane. If she's not dead, why push it? I glare at him, but his arms are crossed. This guy's not going to budge.

"Okay, I choose this one." I point at a big black-bordered ad. It looks depressing enough.

"Good choice." He fills in the blank on his checklist with the funeral home name.

"Now, may I go home?" I ask.

"One more thing. I notice you checked off that Eve is Catholic. Would you like her to receive the 'Sacrament of the Living'?"

I almost choke. The "Sacrament of the Living" is the reformed Catholic Church's watered-down version of the traditional "Last Rites." In the past, Catholics would call a priest to anoint the sick person on his deathbed and to hear a last confession. Very meaningful and comforting. The new version is more priest-friendly. No confession; just a sprinkle of oil. It could be performed at any stage of illness, mostly at the visiting priest's convenience. No more late night calls for them. To me, the "just in case" version is a joke.

However, I am not sure Eve would agree. Perhaps this isn't the time for me to mess around with her spiritual afterlife. Stuffing my personal annoyance with the church's reform, I tell the pastoral director, "Yes, please give her the sacrament. Thank you very much."

Finally, he rises from his chair. We're done! So much for spiritual comfort. As I head for the door, he says, "By the way, my vacation begins tomorrow. I'll be on a cruise for a week. If you need anything, Sister Dorothy will be handling my cases."

Well, okay. "Bon voyage."

The funeral home selection process makes me second-guess my decision to drive home. It's after midnight. Think I'll check out the ICU waiting room. Maybe I'll grab a couple of hours of shut-eye, then go home, feed the cats, and return in time to meet Cass. We can stand watch together through the critical recovery period, whatever that entails.

As I walk into the waiting room, a large fifty-ish woman looks up from the book she's reading. She's munching potato chips. It appears that someone's extended family has populated every couch. Carry-out fried chicken containers dot the coffee tables. There's no place for me except a chair in the corner.

"There's an extra blanket over there," the woman says with a friendly nod. "Looks like my family has taken over all the couches. We're here for my son. He was injured in a motorcycle accident."

"Sorry. How is he?" I ask.

"He's unconscious. Traumatic brain injury. And you?"

"My roommate has a brain aneurysm. She's in surgery."

"Oh, that's too bad. I'll say a prayer for her."

"Thanks. Are you from out of town?"

"No, Green Bay. Haven't been home in four days." She seems proud of the fact, but I wonder why she hasn't been home. Almost anywhere in Green Bay is only 15 minutes from this hospital. Maybe she wants to be close to her son. Well, the poor family doesn't need to catch my bronchitis, too. If I start to cough, I'll wake up all of them. I told the neurosurgeon I was going home, so that's what I'll do.

Shuffling down the corridor, I am overwhelmed by the silence. Is there anything lonelier than an empty hospital late at night?

I've been there before. Fifteen years earlier, my dad had died on the Fourth of July, as fireworks lit up the night sky outside the hospital window. Two years later, my mom's lungs failed on New Year's Eve at midnight. As I helplessly watched her gasp for breath, I asked the nurses to phone the doctor for a knockout drug prescription. Finally, they found him. I could hear the New Year's revelers in the background as the doctor warned me that a drug would send my mom into a final coma. So be it, I had said. The poor woman is out of her mind with panic, drowning in air. In the end, the doctor was right. She slipped into a coma and died 30 hours later.

Where's the damn exit door? Oh, yeah, way down there.

God, I hate hospitals.

# 3

# In a Fog

As I push open the hospital exit door, I'm greeted by a blast of frosty autumn air. I gulp it greedily. The kindly valet appears with an offer to retrieve my car. He doesn't need a description; it's the only car in the lonely lot across the street.

As I wait, I check out the world around me. The stars are still shining, the wind is rustling tree leaves, the moon is playing hide and seek with a cloud. It's amazing: The world the valet lives in hasn't come to an end. I envy him.

He returns in a flash with the car. Refusing my tip with a smile, he gives me directions back to the state highway. Thus I embark on one of the loneliest journeys of my life. From that point to my driveway, 75 miles away, I never see another human—or even a pair of taillights.

It's a straight shot to the Interstate, interrupted only by two or three stoplights. Once I'm on Highway 57, I relax a little. At least I won't get lost. No sooner do I think that thought than a wisp of fog momentarily blurs my vision. Hope that doesn't continue. As I leave the city limits, I flip on my cruise control. "Watch for deer," a sign warns me. It's the last sign I'll see for hours as the fog envelops my car. Damn, I can barely see past the hood. What am I going to do? Better turn back, my good sense suggests. How? I can't see an exit sign. Where are the crossroads? I step on the brakes . . . 60, 40, 20 miles per hour. Even that's too fast, but, gosh darn, I want to get home. Okay, 15 mph. At least, I'll be able to see the deer before I hit it. All right, now. Relax. Take it easy. Just make it home safely. There's a reason for this foggy setback, though I can't fathom what it could be.

Luckily, I'm more tired than sleepy. I say a prayer to the now-defunct Saint Christopher, patron of safe travel. "Dear Saint Christopher, or whoever your replacement is, please get me home safely." I smile at my lame prayer . . . whoa. I slam on the brakes. I can't see diddle, not even the end of my hood. I pray no one's following behind me. No chance of that. Slowly, I pick up the speed, 5, 10, 15 mph again. I wonder if cruise control even works at this speed. Okay, ever onward.

After about ten minutes, I totally forsake the idea of turning around. I'll just aim for staying on pavement. As I drift into a daydream state, the first thought that dances through my head is that Eve and I missed our favorite TV show, *ER*, tonight. I guess we starred in our own drama. And that cute radiologist would've given the *ER* docs a run for their money. What I wouldn't give to have spent a semi-boring night in front of the tube, a cat in each of our laps, and my biggest decision being whether to indulge in a bowl of ice cream or stick to my diet.

Flashing back to my discussion with the neurosurgeon, a thought creeps in. We may never have another routine night. What the hell does a brain aneurysm do to you, anyway? I'm still clueless. Jesus, I hope the surgery goes okay. Please, God, no "I'm sorry" messages on the answering machine. I can't take any more tonight.

"It wasn't supposed to go this way," I shout at the fog. All we wanted was a little piece of the American dream . . . a little art gallery in Door County. Damn, if we had stayed in Naperville, I wouldn't be alone tonight. I'd at least have our A.A. buddies to sit and watch with me. We were stupid to be so adventurous in our fifties. I can hear both of our dead mothers yelling at us for even daring to dream that we could break out of the mundane middle-class way of living.

But really, Mom, what choice did I have? My freelance writing jobs were drying up. Opportunities in the advertising industry were dwindling in Chicago . . . and if anyone was going to get one of the few remaining writing jobs, it wasn't going to be a 51-year-old woman who had blown her career—thanks to alcoholism—15 years before. Even the lower-level jobs I had used as filler between freelance assignments were harder to come by: plum jobs such as lingerie sales-clerk, water meter reader, 800-number operator, shelf-stocker, and the one I dreaded most—cleaning lady. God, I was a lousy cleaning lady. I chuckle as I recall one client screaming at me because I didn't comb the fringe of her living room rug.

Geez, I think I've got a fever, I note, as I squint to see past the headlight glare reflected back at me. My head aches. I'm so tired. Maybe I can amuse myself by trying to figure out where we went wrong. Eve and I had met seven years before at an A.A. meeting. I was working late for one of my west suburban clients and it was time to call it a night. The thought occurred to me that I wouldn't get home in time for my northwest suburban A.A. meeting. No problem; I could make an 8 P.M. meeting in Naperville. It was a plan.

Normally, I'm a little nervous going to an A.A. meeting I've never attended before, but I was pleasantly surprised by the warmth and career orientation of some of the women in the group.

After the meeting, Eve and another lady approached me. "Hi, welcome to the group. I'm Eve, in case you forgot." I looked down at the grinning, short, silver-haired lady before me. She had some spunk about her. "We're all going out now for coffee," she said, "and hot fudge sundaes. Want to join us?"

Well, sure, why not? I needed an A.A. meeting close to work—a place where I could feel comfortable dumping my work frustrations. We headed out for Grandma Sally's, a Naperville coffee shop that welcomed the nightly invasion by one A.A. group or another.

Fortunately, they had a smoking section. (Gotta hang on to one or two addictions in order to feel "alive.")

As I recall our conversation that night, one of the women, an instructor from Northern Illinois University, suggested that we take in a student play that was scheduled for the next Friday. It was an update of a classic Greek tragedy, set in war-torn Bosnia, she explained. Most of the women politely declined. But it sounded weird enough to be fun to me. I had no "life" and the tickets were only five dollars.

"I might go," I piped up.

Eve turned to me, eyes twinkling. "If you'd like to come over to my house after work next Friday, I'll drive us both to De Kalb. Maybe we can squeeze in dinner before the show."

"Sure," I responded. "I'm game." I could use a new A.A. friend, especially one who's intelligent enough to think that seeing a modern day Greek play would be a "hoot."

During the one-hour drive from Naperville through the cornfields to NIU, Eve and I amused ourselves by sharing our stories A.A.-style. That means we tell it the way it was in our drinking days, what happened to bring us into the program, what our lives are like now, and what we hope for in the future.

We discovered that we shared similar semi-strict Catholic upbringings. Though she was a "Southsider," Eve attended Marywood High School in north suburban Evanston. It was a boarding school about three miles away from my parochial high school, Saint Scholastica Academy. Eve was five years older than I, but, interestingly, we both knew some of the same students and teachers.

Eve went on to major in English Lit and Theater Arts at Chicago's Loyola University, and I went south for my advertising communications degree at the University of Illinois in Champaign. Her parents had owned a thriving funeral home business in a Polish neighborhood on Chicago's south side. I figured they had more money than my parents because Eve did her junior year at Loyola's satellite campus in Rome, Italy. I spent my junior year staring out a dorm window at the experimental cornfields across the road.

22

Eve shared how her drinking had escalated after her husband died at the too-young age of 48. It was obvious that she was still very proud of him. He had been a career Army Ranger during the Vietnam War. In fact, she attributed his death from complications from testicular cancer to the fact that he was Agent-Oranged in Vietnam. But that, she said, was hard to prove. It had been seven years since his death, and she was finally ready to think about letting go of her too-big, four-bedroom Naperville house. Her 80-year-old mom, who had been living with her, was happier residing in a nearby fancy residential retirement complex.

"And so, Donna, what's your life like? Advertising's an exciting business, isn't it?"

I replied that maybe real "advertising" was exciting, but not catalog writing. Writing Sears catalogs was my first job out of college. That was followed by many years in business advertising, mainly selling electronics and food. Now *that* was challenging. But since the alcoholism caught up with me, I was back to lowly catalog writing—and damned grateful I had that job.

Eve asked, "So what do you want to do when you retire? What's your dream?"

"Huh? Retire?" Obviously, Eve had no concept of "poor." Between making enough money to pay the bills and going to A.A. meetings, I hardly had time to dream. But why bore her with reality? "Well, since you asked, I guess all I ever really wanted to be was an artist, maybe with my own art gallery, preferably in Door County. That's my impossible dream."

Eve nodded and said, "What an intriguing dream. I used to volunteer at the local arts council. It was fun. Why don't you show me your paintings sometime? Maybe I could represent you. You know, sell your art work to some galleries."

"Uh, that would be great, Eve. But other than a few emergency advertising layouts on the job, I haven't picked up a paintbrush since my last art class 15 years ago. We're discussing hopes here, not realities."

"Oh," she commented, disappointment obvious in her voice. This woman's bored with her life, I thought to myself.

I was right. Over the next year, we became friends. She took a few steps into my world and seemed to enjoy finding cheap or free artsy-type things we could do on a weekend. I appreciated that. During this time, Eve's mom passed away and I helped her walk through her sorrow as best I could.

Soon came an offer I just couldn't refuse. Eve was finally selling her house. Her question was if she bought a Naperville townhouse, did I want to move in with her? Let's see: I lived in a studio apartment in a working-class industrialized area of the so-so suburbs. Eve was talking about luxury living in ultra-chic Naperville. What was the question?

Before I could say "yes," a mental picture of my A.A. sponsor, looking oddly like a "Big Brother" poster, popped into my head.

"Oh wow, Eve. That would really be cool. But only if you figure out a fair-market rent for my room . . . and we split the other stuff."

"Yeah, yeah. Have it your way," Eve grinned. I could see she was not taking me very seriously. I already knew she was generous to a fault.

"I mean it, Eve, or else my sponsor will have my head." There. She could understand that. She had met my A.A. sponsor a few times. Actually, once was enough.

Now I'm crossing the bridge over the canal that joins Lake Michigan and Green Bay in Sturgeon Bay, Door's county seat. All of a sudden, the fog doesn't seem quite as dense. Only 30 to 45 minutes to Baileys Harbor from here, but I'll figure an hour. Who knows what's up ahead?

Now, where was I? Oh yeah, so I moved in with Eve . . . and that was the beginning of our great adventure in free and easy living. Finally, I was able to save some money. Naturally, I wanted to spend it, preferably on a vacation. I hadn't had one in over a decade. We decided on Albuquerque–Santa Fe for our first destination. We so enjoyed the artistic flavor of the Southwest that we set our sights on northern Arizona for the second adventure. We both had dreamed about the sunny high-desert country as a possible relocation option a few years down the road.

By this time, I had become well acquainted with Eve's good friend, Cass, and the three of us did most everything together. Cass couldn't join us on our Arizona trip, but she offered a rather unique way to get a guided tour of our future living options. Call some local Realtors down there, she said. If they're bored, or hungry for new business, they'll show you around town. It's part of their job.

We had a list of five towns we wanted to visit: Prescott, Payson, Cottonwood, Camp Verde, and Sedona, aka Red Rock Country. All of our choices were reasonably affordable, except for incredible Sedona, where we reserved our hotel room. After all, we were on vacation and, besides the Grand Canyon, Sedona was a primo destination.

I was still working 40 hours a week at Spiegel catalog. I briefly debated the wisdom of taking time off when there were rumblings at Spiegel about a major corporate shakeup. I was a freelancer, however, so I didn't really have a job to lose. Meanwhile, lady-of-leisure Eve was planning our itinerary. A couple of days before the trip, she announced that the only Realtor who was interested in Cass's idea was from Sedona.

"Does he understand that we're not multimillionaires?" I asked, remembering photos of Sedona's mansionesque residential dwellings.

"He says he does," Eve shrugged. "I set it up for the second-to-last day. Perhaps we'll be bored and want to see a few luxury ranches."

And so we eventually arrived in drop-dead-gorgeous Sedona. After a week of touring towns that could never compare, we met up with the Realtor in the parking lot of his office. "Okay, what price range are you interested in?" he asked. Eve rattled off the market value of our Naperville townhouse, while I nonchalantly added that I was only interested in a house with one of the awesome Red Rock views. Eve and I exchanged smug smiles in the back of the car, knowing there was no way we could afford Sedona, so we would just enjoy the tour.

We figured the Realtor knew that at some level but didn't have anything better to do the first week of December. We were barely paying attention to his chatter when we realized that he was saying, "I've got a perfect three-bedroom ranch I want you to see, three miles down the road. It has wonderful Red Rock views." He was right; Eve bought it in a "bliss blackout" the next day. Four months later, we moved to paradise.

I had brought along a couple of little freelance accounts, but Eve had been emphatic that I had a new direction. "Go learn to be an artist," she commanded. "I'll carry us financially for a couple of years. Maybe we'll set up a gallery, or maybe we'll just sell to them. If you're worried about your pride, sell your car. We'll just use mine, and you can throw that money into the pot. Let me manage the finances while you paint."

I tried to tell her that I didn't think I had enough talent; but she really liked my art style, so there was nothing to talk about. Nobody had ever believed in me like that. I said I would try my best.

Two and a half years later, I was selling a painting here and there . . . but I was still a ways from big-time gallery appeal. Meanwhile, our social life was primarily built around A.A., which isn't bad except that most Sedona meetings were infected by the kissy-huggy style from that land to the west, where many A.A. groups were little more than social clubs.

Truth be told, I missed the occasional miserable Midwest overcast day. And it appeared that Eve had descended into a funky depression mode. From my viewpoint, she was addicted to the Internet . . . and once a month she did battle with a whopper migraine headache. Though she denied unhappiness, I figured she missed her multitude of friends in Chicago. I pushed hard a suggestion to move back and, finally, she relented. I had heard around the A.A. tables the folly of the "geographic" cure. I thought our case was different, but Eve's headaches and depression continued.

Meanwhile, I scrambled to find some freelance accounts. We were living in a rented condo in Naperville and shopping around for a townhouse. We had been back almost nine months when we decided to take a break and head up to Door County, Wisconsin, for a three-day weekend.

We had promised each other we wouldn't look at real estate on this trip. We already knew we couldn't afford the lakefront home I always dreamed of, and anything else seemed unbearable to me. Anyway, the entire county job market was based on tourism, and though Eve didn't discuss finances with me, I knew the move from Sedona had cost us dearly.

# In a Fog

It was a rainy spring weekend in Door County. I took off for the state park to take photos of wildflowers in between the showers. Eve said she wanted to walk around Baileys Harbor and browse the shops. The way she told it, a cloudburst sent her scurrying into a Realtor's office for shelter. While she was waiting, she thumbed through a February home listing guide. There on page 33 was a modest ranch house boasting 100 feet of shoreline, listed at the price of our Sedona house.

As it turned out, the house was owned by a Realtor I had known from my family excursions to Door County as a teenager. Two days later, Eve bought the house. I wasn't sure if she was completely crazy, but I would hardly ever object to her buying my dream home on the lake.

Surprise, surprise. The 50-year-old house had quite a few more faults than the building inspection report revealed. For example, the bathroom floor was rotting under the tub. Thirty thousand dollars in necessary improvements forced Eve to take out a loan, a five-year mortgage we would pay back by getting jobs, but not until the next summer.

Now I'm rounding the bend that offers a panoramic view of the Lake and Baileys Harbor in the daylight. Oh, boy. Daylight, I ruefully note, is only two hours away. And then I have to slam on the brakes again. There, in the middle of the highway in town, are three deer standing at attention, transfixed by my headlights. "Oh, go away," I mutter exhaustedly. Surprisingly, they do—but they sure take their sweet time about it.

While I wait, I take the opportunity to thank all the higher-powers-that-be for my safe trip. I continue to pray all the way to my driveway, out of the car, and into the house. Oh, no—the answering machine is blinking. I tentatively touch the button. Thank God, it's only Cass, confirming her departure time of 6 A.M. That's only two hours from now. God, I'm tired—sick, too. I fall into bed, and a fitful sleep follows.

# 4

# Coma—Prognosis Unknown

"Ouch, Lola, that's my toe you're biting. What the . . . ?" Oh. Apparently the alarm clock has been ringing for ten minutes. No wonder the cat's crazed. Then it dawns on me. Last night was not good; today may be worse.

Up in a flash, I stumble down the hallway, bypassing the bathroom, and head for the answering machine in the dining room. It's blinking. I close my eyes and press the button. It's the brain surgeon. "Good news. The operation was a success. But the next 48 hours are critical." He promises to keep an eye on Eve's progress and check on her later, but he probably won't talk to me again until tomorrow.

Okay. That's a relief. I must have been out of it last night. Usually, a ringing phone awakens me. The next message is Cass, saying she's leaving Naperville at 6:30 A.M. I better get going or I'll be late for our meeting.

Suddenly, I realize how lousy I feel. Nevertheless I race

through dressing and feeding the cats. No time for breakfast—not hungry anyway.

Before I depart, I make a quick call to Cass to give her directions to the hospital. Then I call my local G.P. His nurse takes my message. "Hi, Carol. I know the doctor never prescribes medication over the phone, but I'm certain I have bronchitis and my roommate is in the ICU in Green Bay. I can't come in for a checkup, but I need a prescription for something to knock this thing out. They won't let me into ICU if I look as sick as I feel. Please help me."

Carol promises to beg the doctor on my behalf and let me know what happens. Darn, I almost had this thing beat on my own. Oh-oh, better check the food supply. Gosh, I hope Cass doesn't make me cook dinner for her. What's this? Chicken? How old is that? Oh, yeah, Eve promised to make fried chicken last night. Rats, I wish I hadn't looked. Misty-eyed, I close the fridge and pick up meowing Lola, who wants a hug. I need one, too. I gotta get out of here.

Can you believe it? It's another gorgeous day. I whiz past golden pastures, blazing trees, and russet-red barns, under an impossibly blue sky. Heading down Highway 57, I note there's no fog to obscure my view of the bay through the trees. It's more blue than green today.

I arrive at the hospital with enough time to check in at the ICU before Cass arrives. I head up. The elevator doors open, but the ICU door is closed and locked tight. A posted sign discourages visitors before 10 A.M. Oh, screw it.

I head for the neuro-ICU waiting room, where a party is obviously in progress. I plop down in front of a TV. Cartoons. Oh, brother. As I thumb through a *People* magazine, I can't help listening in on the goings-on. They're loud.

"Hi, Russ. Hi, Frank."

"How's it going, Fran? Where's Nancy?"

"Out for donuts."

"Got any Fritos?"

"Hey, Frank, grab that remote, willya?"

Presto. The cartoons are replaced by Eeeeee-ow. Eeeeee-ow.

Formula One racing on ESPN. Whoopee. Eeeeee-ow. I gotta get out of here.

Outside, I notice signs posted by the doors forbidding smoking on hospital property. So fine. Screw you. I'll go home. You'd think they'd encourage it. There are big bucks in the diseases caused by smoking. I note that I'm in a surly mood.

"Donna! Donna!" It's Cass, emerging from the parking area.

"Cass, what are you doing here already? What did you do, fly?"

"Three and a half hours door-to-door. Thank God for radar detectors. How's Eve?"

"She survived the surgery."

Immediately, Cass' face brightens, and then the tears start to flow. "I was so scared to ask that question. It did not sound good last night, you know. I packed my black dress, just in case."

"We're not out of the woods yet, Cass. The next 48 hours will be critical, according to the surgeon. But don't ask me what they expect could go wrong. I haven't a clue. Well, by my watch, ICU is open now. Let's go see Eve."

Inside ICU, I nudge Cass and direct her toward their main desk. Naturally, none of the nurses look familiar. It's a new shift.

"Hi, Donna Siles here to see Eve. And can I talk to her nurse, please, to find out how she's doing?"

The desk nurse brings out her clipboard and checks it. "Sorry," she says. "I don't have your name on my list. Are you a blood relative?"

"No, I am not. But I am her power of attorney—and what do you mean I'm not on the list? Who do you think filled out the admission forms last night?"

She shrugs. "Sorry, you're not a blood relative; you'll have to go down to patient services and talk to them."

I can feel my face flush. Anger is bubbling up. I'm on a fast track to rage. "I'm not going down to your patient services. I am waiting right here for you to check this out." I'm sputtering now.

Ever the diplomat, Cass worms herself in between the desk and me. "What she means," Cass sweetly drawls, "is that there's obviously been a mix-up. Perhaps you can check, and we'll go sit in the visiting area and wait for you to come get us. By the way, I'm Cass Davis from Chicago. I know I'm not on the list, but Eve has no blood relatives within 300 miles. We are her best friends."

The nurse stops glaring at me long enough to give Cass a warm smile. "That's a good idea. This will only take about ten minutes. I'll find you."

I want to slug her, but Cass shoves me back and toward the exit door. Out of the corner of my eye, I see Eve in her little room. Looks like she's sleeping, I hope. Damn, I'm angry.

Once out the door, Cass admonishes me. "For heaven's sake, Donna, don't alienate the nurses. You need them. It's just a little mix-up. Calm down. Hey, you don't look so well. You sick, honey?"

"Hmmphf." I spin away from Cass's friendly touch. "You know, Cass, I could have been sitting in that waiting room all night . . . probably until doomsday. What if Eve had died during the operation? They obviously didn't even know I existed. How could they come and get me?"

"But Eve didn't die. And we're grateful for that, aren't we? I'm telling you again, calm down. Here. Let's go sit in the visitor's room."

"You don't want to do that, Cass. I'm warning you."

"Don't be silly. Come on."

We find a sofa and plop down. I can hardly hide my smirk, as Cass acclimates herself to the environment. Eeee-ow.

"What the hell is that?" Cass asks.

"ESPN . . . in stereo, I believe."

"Let's get the hell out of here. We'll go stand by ICU. Better yet, where's the bathroom? It's been hours for me, and you need to splash some cold water on your wrists. Cool down. Come on."

After the bathroom break, we return to the corridor outside the waiting area. I can view the "party" from there, through the windows, without the sound effects. I use this opportunity to exercise one of my personality flaws: judgmentalism. Yep, judging from the leather garb, these must be friends of the guy who injured himself in a motorcycle accident.

Shouldn't they be at work or something? I wonder. They look a little scruffy. I'll bet . . . uh-oh, my 12-Step program kicks in. "You're supposed to bless this motorcycle gang, Donna," my program voice says. "You can't afford any resentments or any anger this morning. And, while you're at it, bless that ICU nurse and the whole hospital staff."

Just then, the nurse appears. After a quick smile for Cass, she coolly addresses me, "We're sorry for the mix-up. There was a crisis up here in the ICU last night. In the confusion, your name didn't make it onto the clipboard. Both of you are on the list now. By the way, what is your cell phone number?"

"I don't have one," I announce proudly, then realize that this young nurse couldn't possibly relate to my point of pride.

But Cass gets it, and I'm sure she doesn't like it. She quickly says, "I'll give you my cell number. I'll be with Donna for at least four days. Somebody's got to calm her down." Grin.

I note that the warm fuzzies are flying between those two again. Oh, screw it . . . or bless it . . . or whatever.

Finally, we're following the nurse into ICU and Eve's little room. Sure looks like a lot of "life support" is going on. As if she's reading my mind, the nurse says, "The only life support Eve is hooked up to is the ventilator. The doctor thinks this is best for postsurgical recovery. Her brain doesn't have to work at helping her breathe; it can concentrate on healing.

"As you can see, Eve is resting comfortably. She is stable; her condition is as expected. We prefer that you do not stimulate her with talking or touching. Please limit this visit to ten minutes. You may then return in three hours and visit again for ten minutes."

The nurse departs. I realize I've been avoiding looking at Eve until now. Cass speaks up. "Well, I don't care what she says," she announces defiantly. "I drove up from Chicago to see my friend and I'm gonna give her a kiss." When she bends down to kiss Eve's cheek, Eve's eyes fly open . . . and, hey, is that a smile for Cass?

"My turn," I say. Gingerly, I peck at Eve's cheek. I wait. No response. "Oh, it just figures," I mutter.

"Oh, you know she knows you're here," Cass says cheerily.

No, I don't know that. But, okay, if it makes Cass feel better to say it, I'll go along.

"Geez, she looks so tiny," Cass comments. "And look at that huge bandage on her head."

Oh, I'm looking all right; it's making me sick. I turn my attention to the monitors. "Do you know what they're measuring, Cass?"

Just then, the nurse pops in and gives the monitors an eye. "Time's up, folks," she says. "Eve's stimulated by your presence. Her blood pressure is on the rise."

Guess I can't argue with that. Heads down, we shuffle out like two naughty schoolgirls ejected from our classroom. I can't resist a parting shot. "Bye, Eve, we'll be back at two." There, now I feel better.

"Well, what are we going to do for three hours, besides go out for a cigarette right now?" I ask. "We're going to get awfully sick of each other's company, I fear. I know how I get on your nerves when Eve's not around to act as a buffer between us, Cass."

"That's not going to happen," Cass replies as we head toward the elevators. "I was thinking all the way up here about the weird conversation I had with Eve the last time she was in to visit with me."

"Oh, yeah? What was that?"

The elevator door opens and we're facing a crowd of bubbling, smiling young people holding stuffed animals and flowers. There ought to be a law against happy maternity visitors traveling on the same elevators with ICU visitors. Cass and I quietly board and shrink into our respective corners for the ride down.

The glee is almost more than I can bear. When we hit the first floor, Cass and I take the lead in a race to the door. The chill of the brisk autumn day embraces us as we exit.

While we fidget with our lighters and cigarettes in the breeze, Cass relates her month-ago conversation with Eve. "As I was saying, it was really weird. Has Eve been complaining of bad headaches or any symptoms that would lead to this aneurysm?"

I shake my head. "No, nothing. No recent migraines, either." I wonder what Cass is driving at.

"Well, Eve and I were having coffee one morning and, from out of the blue, Eve says, "If anything happens to me, Cass, would you promise me to watch out for Donna? You know, I wouldn't want her to get so upset that she'd drink or something."

My mouth drops open. That's so unlike Eve to talk that way. Cass pauses to appreciate my reaction.

"Well, I was stunned," Cass drawls. "I asked Eve if she was sick and hadn't told you. But, no, Eve said she was okay. She just insisted that I make this promise. I said, well, of course, I'd do anything for her. Then the conversation ended with one of our usual jokes about your dramatics. And I forgot all about it, until today."

"That sure is weird, Cass. It's not like Eve to even pretend to be psychic . . . or to talk that seriously, for that matter."

Cass says, "Well, I'm going to ask her what that was all about when she wakes up. Gave me the willies today. Anyway, it all means that we're not going to argue or fight while I am here." Cass crushes her cigarette butt and—with no ashtray in sight—tosses it in the street. I, being the environmentally conscious good girl, pocket my butt. I note there are two other butts already in that pocket. Pretty soon, I'm going to stink. Oh, well . . .

"Shall we see what delicious items the hospital cafeteria is offering for lunch? I'm starved," Cass says as she turns to head off.

"I'm not a bit hungry," I mutter to myself, as I follow her down the sidewalk. Then I remember how comforting a hospital toasted cheese sandwich was when I was doing the last-days vigil with my parents. Gotta eat something; maybe I can get up for that.

"What? No toasted cheese sandwich on the menu in a Wisconsin hospital cafeteria? And—hey—it's Friday and this place is Catholic. Oh, for crying out loud," I sputter.

Cass is now eyeing me seriously to see if I might have stepped over the edge.

"Never mind," I say, holding up my hand in an effort to halt ANY concerned comment. "I'll calm down, starting now. The hot dogs look delicious."

The rest of the lunch is uneventful, and rather tasteless. I believe that hot dog is going to come back and cause some trouble. I won't do that again.

Finally, it's two o'clock. We find our way back to ICU and this time the reception nurse welcomes us with a nod. "Eve's resting; don't stimulate her," she calls after us as we enter Eve's darkened room. This time we obey. After 15 minutes of staring at Eve, the monitors, and each other, Cass yawns. Then I yawn.

I speak. "Unless you have an objection, Cass, I think we should head back home after this. I don't feel so great and you must be bushed from the drive. If we stay for the five o'clock visiting session, we'll be traveling during "deer on the road" time. Or, worse yet, the fog will come in. I'll tell the nurse that we'll call in at six o'clock and she's to let us know if there is a change. Okay?"

"Good idea," Cass agrees. "Nothing we can do here." We rise from our hard wooden visitors' chairs in unison and bid good-night to Eve. Then Cass catches my eye as I catch hers. Quickly, furtively, we each sneak a peck on Eve's cheek . . . and then hastily retreat before the alarms go off.

On the way out, we walk past the visitor's room as a group of couples gather at the door, loaded down with carry-out chicken and pizza. With the door open, a screaming Eeeeee-ow escapes.

Cass asks, "Is that damned race still going on?"

"Don't know, don't care. We're out of here," I respond as we quicken our pace to the elevators.

Cass insists that I leave my car in the hospital parking lot and that she will drive home. (Hmmm, guess I'm not behaving too rationally.) I don't argue with her.

The trip is happily uneventful and—thanks to Cass's radar detector—quite speedy. Very quiet, too, except for Cass's calls home to check on her work situation and the cat's well-being. Back home, there's a message on the answering machine that super-meds for my bronchitis are waiting for me at a Sturgeon Bay pharmacy. We can stop on the way to the hospital Saturday morning. Next, I give our cats an update on "Auntie Eve" as I prepare their dinners. Cass has found a bag of potato chips in the cupboard. She's happily munching as she takes the chicken out of the refrigerator and announces that she will fix dinner! Thank you, God. I readily agree to her conditions: that she will cook dinners while she is here, but I must do the dishes. Sounds like a deal to me. And, oh yeah, don't come near her when she's in the kitchen. Fat chance of that.

I meekly mention that I'm not very hungry, not wanting to offend a gourmet chef. Cass replies, "Have I ever fixed a meal that you and Eve haven't inhaled? I guarantee you'll eat this. Where's the Campbell's soup?"

While Cass does her thing, I hunt for fresh linens to make up her bed. We'll be lucky to stay awake until eight o'clock.

"Dinnertime," she calls out. Wow, it sure doesn't look like chicken and soup. "What did you do to this?" I ask, as I shovel one forkful after another into my mouth. "You're a gourmet genius, Cass."

"It's easy, simple. I'll teach you because you'll probably be doing the cooking for a while." I graciously accept her offer while I mentally review my mind-file of "edible" frozen dinners, from my days before Eve's cooking.

After dinner and doing dishes, we make a few more phone calls. A call to the hospital is rewarded with relatively good news: Eve's condition is stable. She's resting comfortably. My final call is to Eve's cousin, Vivian. I haven't talked to her yet and I need to remind her to sign the power of attorney document the hospital is sending her.

"How is Eve?" Vivian asks.

She sounds concerned, so I tell her all the details, ending with the doctor's 48-hour critical watch statement.

She responds, "Well, next week Steve and I are going on vacation. Taking the camper. Hope that hospital thing arrives on Monday because at 6 A.M. Tuesday we'll be on our way. We're looking forward to it. Gosh, I sure hope Eve doesn't die while I'm gone."

I'm floored. I know my mouth is wide open because Cass is staring at me. "Okay, Vivian," I stutter into the phone, "you have a good time. Could you just give me a call on Monday to let me know about the power of attorney document? I'd appreciate it. Thanks."

I drop the receiver onto the cradle. Turning to Cass, I realize I can't speak. Finally, the words tumble out.

Cass's mouth drops open. "Eve's always giving her something. I can't believe it. You must have said something wrong to her."

"I didn't," I protest. "You heard me. I just told her what happened to Eve. Nothing about me. I don't get it. Oh yeah, I guess I do. I'm remembering some people's weird reactions to my phone calls that my Mom was near the end. One of her best friends couldn't "make it" to the funeral. I figured then that it was because Mom was relatively young, only 63. Maybe Mom's friends couldn't face the wake-up call that all of us are mortal."

"Forget it," Cass says. "This is not good talk before bed. We've got to get our sleep so that we can be there for Eve. Don't think so much. Bless her cousin and be done with it."

I am so tired I don't even want to argue with Cass. We both shut up and go to bed.

Next morning, before we take off for the hospital, Cass suggests we take along an ice chest. "Maybe we can do some grocery shopping in Green Bay." Then Cass confesses, "I ate most of the potato chips, and I needed a midnight snack of cookies and milk. No more cookies," she adds, not the least bit apologetically.

Cass speeds us to Green Bay while I try hard to keep my mind on the scenery rather than the day ahead. When we walk into ICU, we're greeted by a friendly nurse who actually smiles at me, too.

She says, "Eve's awake now and I was just about to go in to ask her the routine questions. Would you like to join me?"

Cass and I nod enthusiastically. Following the nurse, we elbow each other gleefully.

"She's awake! She's awake!" I chant in Cass's ear.

And there's Eve, sitting up in bed. "Hi," Eve whispers to Cass. Eve is smiling broadly.

"Okay, Eve," the nurse says, as she assumes control. "I am going to ask you some questions. Ready? What's your first name?"

"Eve."

"And your last name?"

"Kasper."

"Good. Now, Eve, where do you live?"

"Baileys Harbor," she says hoarsely.

"Doing well. Do you know what day it is?"

"Friday?" Eve mouths.

The nurse shakes her head.

"Saturday?" Eve grins sheepishly as the nurse pats her.

"Good, Eve. Now, how old are you?"

Eve looks at her blankly.

"Um, 43?"

"You wish," Cass blurts out.

"Shhh," the nurse says. "No, Eve, you're 55. But that's all for now. You did pretty darned good, Eve."

The nurse smiles at us, nods, and departs. Part of me wants to celebrate with Eve and the other part wants to follow that nurse and make her tell me why Eve thinks she's 43. I opt for the celebration.

Cass beats me to Eve. When she's done hugging and kissing, I take my turn. I'm so pleased I think I will melt.

"What happened?" Eve asks, pointing at her head.

I'm just about to launch into the story when the nurse returns to eject us.

"She needs to rest now," the nurse explains. "Say your good-byes. You can visit again around three o'clock."

While the nurse stands there, we quickly pat Eve on the arm and tell her, "Hang in there. We'll be back."

Cass and I are just too jubilant. "Let's go for breakfast somewhere to celebrate," Cass says. "Then we'll shop for cookies and stuff."

Sounds like a plan to me and off we go. Halfway through breakfast, I'm visited by a nagging feeling of doom. What's that about, I wonder? Maybe it's Eve's age question.

"Cass, what do you think Eve's answer of 43 means?"

"Oh, I don't know. Probably nothing," she dismisses my anxiety. "For Pete's sake, the woman just had brain surgery. You think too much, Donna. Lighten up."

Maybe Cass is right. I'll just shut up and enjoy the good news. I shake my doubts as Cass and I go searching for a grocery store. Cass loads up the cart with junk food while I ponder the variety of teas. Though I managed two meals in a row, I have serious doubts about my tummy's continued cooperation in the digestion process.

We take the groceries out to the car, then return to visit the mini shopping mall next door. We both lose track of time browsing in a bookstore, until Cass remembers to check her watch. "Better get back," she says. "It's almost three o'clock. We don't want them to deny us entry."

Still giddy with the morning's glad tidings, we rumble through the ICU doors. I'm heading toward Eve's room past the reception desk when I'm stopped short by the morning nurse's cold, icy stare.

"What's the matter?" I squeak.

"Where were you?" she asks. "We looked for you everywhere. We tried calling your home." She glares at Cass. "We tried your cell phone, your office, your home."

"What's the matter?" I plead for an answer.

"Eve postured," the nurse says flatly.

"I don't understand. She did what?"

"She postured. She was dying. Like dead. We had to rush her into surgery. We needed your consent."

"Well, did she die? Where is she? What happened? We just went out for food." I'm squeaking again.

"Eve came back from surgery with Dr. Brum about ten minutes ago. She's alive, but she's in a coma. You should have told us you were leaving the hospital. Here. Sign this consent form now. I'll page Dr. Brum for you. I don't know if he's still in the hospital."

I look over at Cass. She's holding her cell phone, staring at it in dumb disbelief. "It was on," she's mumbling. "I don't understand. It was on."

I finish signing the form. The nurse hands me her phone. It's Dr. Brum.

"What happened, doctor?" I ask.

"I don't know. She was doing so well. Don't know what happened. But she was dying. We had to give her a chance, right? She is so young. I know your wishes, but we had to try. We put in a valve.

Did you see it? Do you understand? We had to relieve the pressure on her brain. She's in a coma now. All we can do is wait and see. I'll be in the hospital tomorrow. I'll meet you by the visiting room at one o'clock. We'll talk then. Understand?"

"I guess so," I say.

"Good. See you tomorrow. You take it easy. Nothing we can do but wait and see."

I hand the phone back to the nurse. She glares at me again. "We tried to find you," she says, shaking her head and turning away. "Oh," she adds, "you can see Eve. But just for a minute."

"Thank you," Cass and I mutter as we make our way to Eve's room. It's dark in here. Eve's face is lighted by the glow of instrument panels. She looks almost angelic . . . and very dead to the bleeping world around her.

I can see tears streaming down Cass' cheeks as she bends over Eve to kiss her. I'm way beyond tears. My stomach is lurching. Please, God, I don't want to be sick in here. I bend over Eve. Cass was right; she seems so tiny. "I am so sorry I wasn't here for you," I whisper. And now the tears come.

"I've got to get out of here, Cass. Please, I don't want to lose it in here."

Cass grabs me and hugs me for dear life. We back out of the door, as if we can't bear to turn our backs on Eve again.

The atmosphere in this ICU is frigid, as a couple of nurses look up and scowl at our retreat. Heads bowed, Cass and I walk toward the exit. Nobody says good-bye.

# 5

# "Vegetable"

Saturday night is filled with fear and tears, "if onlys" and "buts."
On Sunday, Cass and I meet with the neurosurgeon, Dr. Brum,
at the appointed hour. He takes a minute to update Cass.

"Eve suffered a level-five brain aneurysm Thursday. That, combined with the grand mal seizure, created a life-threatening condition. I operated that night to clip the aneurysm. The surgery was
successful. The patient's recovery was going well until Saturday afternoon. A sudden fluid buildup exerted pressure on the brain, requiring emergency surgery to relieve the pressure to save her life."

Turning to me, he says, "We don't know why that happened, but
she is unconscious now. Since you weren't here to consent to the surgery, I based my decision on our conversation Thursday night. We
had to give her a chance, right?"

I believe the man's eyes are misty with emotion. No doubt, he did
what he thought best. I do trust him.

He continues. "But, now, all we can do is wait. Hopefully, we will know more about her condition by next weekend. There's nothing you can do."

But pray, I add to myself. Pray for what? I do not know. The 12-Step program is so ingrained in me that I long ago gave up on praying for an outcome of my choosing. Instead, I pray for acceptance of life on life's terms, and the strength to act accordingly.

Codependently enough, I find myself saying consoling words to the doctor. Simultaneously, I'm trying to make myself believe that I can actually walk through the week and leave the outcome up to God, without overthinking medical strategies I know nothing about.

Before he departs, I ask the doctor if he will accept a call midweek from another of Eve's cousins, a physician in St. Louis. I know he is fond of Eve and my thinking is that he can interpret the medical facts in a way I can understand the situation better. Dr. Brum readily agrees. Then he's gone, and Cass and I are left standing there to stare at each other.

"Let's see if the new shift of nurses will let us in to see Eve," Cass wryly suggests. Why not? So off we go for another uneventful visit with our comatose friend.

Later that evening, I make some more phone calls, including one to Eve's physician cousin. After he agrees to call the neurosurgeon, he relates the story about one of his physician friends who had spent many years caring for his post–brain aneurysm vegetable wife. This doctor employed a paid caretaker by day and attended to her at night. The woman had finally died, which—I gather from the tone—was a blessing for all.

That phone call is followed by one to Eve's late husband's sister, Arlene, and her husband, Jim. They offer some helpful suggestions on communicating with an unconscious patient. They should know. They are in their eighth year of caregiving their adult son who suffered traumatic brain injury in an auto accident.

After I hang up, I turn to Cass, "Guess I'm not the only one in the world with problems." That insight keeps me from feeling sorry for myself for the rest of the night.

Monday morning, Cass orders me to stay home, preferably in

bed, to hasten my recovery from the bronchitis. "I'll drive to Green Bay for the next couple of days. On Wednesday, I'll stop at the hospital but then head back to Chicago. I need to go to work and you need to get well, to handle this routine on your own."

That inspires a pitiful coughing fit from me. How manipulative can one be? Gosh, I don't want to be alone. Ever-cool Cass simply raises an eyebrow to warn me not to try that ploy again.

"You can spend Wednesday cleaning up the mess I've made," Cass says, unable to resist the dig. "Perhaps today you could glance at Eve's insurance policy to see exactly what it will cover, then report back to me so I'm sure you understand. Okay?"

"You're so right," I say. Now that's the kind of friend I need in a crisis. We both know that if I allow myself to go down emotionally, it's a long, hard trip back up to the level of normal functioning. I can't afford self-pity now.

The next couple of days proceed according to Cass's plan. Together we make sense of the insurance policy, and I receive a lesson in the pitfalls of catastrophic coverage. "Hmmm. No matter how I read this," Cass says, "it still comes out the same. Eve is entitled to a whopping 12 days of nursing home coverage."

I respond. "Well, let's hope we don't have to go there. Why look for trouble we don't have yet?"

"Most people try to plan to avoid trouble, Donna, but not you two Pollyannas."

I cringe at the shot. Can't argue with the truth.

"Anyway," she says, "the good news is they'll cover that month of in-hospital rehabilitation that Eve's surgeon told you about. Maybe you can ask Eve's cousin to explain that to you."

Good idea. He had promised to call the surgeon the next day and get back to me that night.

"One final sticky point about this wonderful insurance coverage of Eve's. You do realize that the $5,000 deductible goes into effect again at the beginning of the next calendar year? You better pray that Eve's out of the hospital by December 31. That's less than two and a half months away."

Her words make me realize I am secretly expecting Eve to snap out of her coma this weekend and be back on her merry way to health. Absolutely no one has alluded to that sort of outcome since Saturday's debacle.

"Uh-oh," I respond. What else can I say?

Cass bids farewell to me on Wednesday morning. "I'm concerned about you," she says. "You still look a little sick, or maybe it's shell shock. Keep busy with the mundane tasks today. Do two loads of laundry, mop a floor. I'll call you when I get home. I'll expect you to tell me that you functioned all day. Deal?"

"Sure, Cass." I can barely conceal my fear of the day ahead. Will I function, I wonder?

Surprise. I do. Knowing that Cass will call motivates me through the day. Slowly, my shaken confidence is returning. I really don't understand why an event beyond my control would destroy my confidence in the first place. But it has.

That evening I enjoy the leftovers from one of Cass's meals. I toss the final load of laundry into the washing machine and amuse myself with computer solitaire. I promised Eve's sister-in-law, Arlene, that I would wait at least a week before I went sleuthing online for brain aneurysm facts. I agreed with her that the addictive action of searching might shove my brain into "information overload."

Anyway, I am hoping for enlightenment from Eve's physician cousin. I anxiously anticipate his phone call. Any minute now, I say to myself as I eye the clock. It's 7 P.M.

Solitaire. Hearts. Free Cell. I've played them all tonight. Now it's approaching 10 P.M. I called Eve's cousin at 8 P.M., but all I got was an answering machine. Man, where is he? He promised. The combination of anxiety and super-drugs is making me sleepy.

R-R-Ring! The jangle of the telephone shoots me to the ceiling. It's 11 P.M.

"Hello? Dave?" I say tentatively. Yes, it's him all right.

"You blew it," he growls. His anger and frustration fill my ear. "You should have pulled the plug when you had the chance. Now you're stuck with a hopeless vegetable."

At first, I'm speechless. Then I protest, "But I never had the opportunity to pull the plug. I told them no extraordinary measures. But I wasn't there and . . ." Oh, hell, what's the use? "What can I do now?" I whimper.

"Pray for pneumonia," he says, "then pull the plug."

Huh? What is this man saying? I know he loves Eve. "What happens if I can't do that?" I ask, knowing already that I don't want to hear the answer.

"You will be caregiving a vegetable for the rest of your life—or Eve's. If it was difficult for my wealthy doctor friend, it's impossible for you. What kind of nursing home coverage does Eve have?"

"Next to none," I respond. My voice is trembling. In fact, just about every body part is shaking to some degree.

"Then you'll have to dissolve all of Eve's assets and put her on Medicaid. Luckily, you two own the house jointly, right?"

I am going to throw up. "Actually, no," I say. "I sold my half back to Eve for a dollar six months ago. It made getting the mortgage an easier process. It was all very legal, a quitclaim deed thing with a lawyer. I feel sick."

"Yeah, you don't sound so good. The wife and I plan to come up and see Eve the weekend after next. See you then. Better get to bed now . . . and think about what I've said. Refuse treatment for pneumonia. Good night, now." He signs off.

I am sick. In a daze, I travel from the dining room to the bathroom to the bedroom. I turn out the lights and collapse into bed. My brain is audibly buzzing. The head noise intermingles with the sound of the lake through the open window. I listen.

Waves are rolling in, splashing the rocks along the shore. In . . . out. In . . . out. The lake's siren song is calling me. "Come on in. I'll carry you out and away from all your woes." In . . . out.

"Stop it," I yell, startling the cats at the foot of the bed. Their eyes are glowing in the moonlight. In . . . out. Are the waves getting louder?

"Damn it, please die, Eve! Make her die, God." Christ, I can't pray that prayer. What am I going to do? I can't caregive a vegetable for the rest of my life. This is too much, God. I can't. Please, let me die, instead. Take me now.

In . . . out. I'm sitting on the edge of the bed now, holding on to my head. Got to keep my mind inside my head, but it keeps leaking out and floating toward the window. In . . . out. Stop it. Try and think of something. I do, but as quickly as a thought comes, it slithers away. I just can't hold on to it. Maybe I'll try praying.

"Mom?" I pray. "Please help me."

No response.

"Jesus, Mary, Joseph, God?"

No response.

"Mommy?" I try again. No? Well then, how about Eve's mom? "Sophie? Are you there? Yes?" Yes, I think she is. "Hey, listen to me. Dave said I've got to pray for pneumonia . . . and I will," I threaten her. "So if you want your daughter to live, you better help me save my mind tonight. I think I'm having a breakdown. I don't know, I've never had one. But Eve isn't going to make it very well without me. You've got to help me make it through the night. PLEASE."

I feel a smidgen of calmness. Get up, have a cup of tea, a voice says inside my head. Okay. I obey. Yes, I can walk down this hall. Yes, I can heat water in the microwave. Yes, I can taste the tea. I'll just sit here at the dining room table until dawn comes. Got to hold on to my mind until 5 A.M. Then I can call Cass. Yes. That's what I'll do. I lay my poor head on a place mat and drift off into the twilight zone.

# 6

# Seek, Knock, Ask

First light rouses me. I can call Cass in a few minutes. I'm still here. I'm okay. I'm freezing to death. I retrieve two blankets from the bedroom and wrap myself up. I can't stop shivering. God, my teeth are chattering.

Finally, 5 A.M. I call Cass. She picks up.

"I'm sorry to wake you, Cass. But Dave, Eve's cousin, called last night." I relate the conversation.

"He's crazy," Cass screams into my ear. "Who the hell does he think he is? God? He had no right to say that to you. No right at all. Damn. Why didn't he call before I left? He's off his rocker, Donna. Listen to me. You heard—I heard—the surgeon say to wait until this weekend. We will know more then. That's what you are going to do. Do you understand? Wait. That's all you have to do." Cass pauses. "Donna? You there? Say something."

"I'm very cold. Very tired, Cass. But thank you. You're right. I'll just wait. Wish I'd stop shaking . . . Cass, I'm afraid."

"Well, sure you are; you're dealing with Eve's coma."

"But that's not all, Cass."

"What else is bothering you?"

"The house. We're going to lose it. The government will take it away for Medicaid. How else can I pay for Eve's nursing home?"

"That's ridiculous, Donna. You own that house, too."

"No, I don't, Cass. I sold my share to Eve."

"Oh no! What weed were you two smoking? Well, you're not budging from that house. Tell you what. I'll be talking to my lawyer friend today anyway. I'll ask his opinion. Promise me you won't think about that until I call you back. I'm really busy. You won't hear from me until 4 or 5 P.M. And, Donna, do not go to the hospital today. Stay home and sleep. Promise?"

"Okay."

"When you wake up, I want you to dust the living room, please. Vacuum, too. It really needs it. I dropped a lot of cookie crumbs."

I giggle.

"That-a-girl. Call your sponsor this morning. Maybe she'll yell at you. You deserve it. Talk to you later."

Half an hour after hanging up with Cass, I realize that I haven't moved from the dining room table. What have I been doing? I can't recall my thoughts. My brain is buzzing. Did I fall asleep? I don't think so. Did I black out? Maybe. God, that's dangerous territory, Donna. Stand up, I order myself. Did I feed the cats? Their bowls are empty. I don't know. Big fat Ozzie could have eaten it all. Both he and Lola are pacing. I think they're giving me dirty looks. Oh hell, I can't remember. Just play it safe and feed them again. Move, Donna.

Okay, that's done. Now I better eat. I can't. I'm not hungry. You must eat, I argue. Opening the refrigerator, I pray something will look appealing. There. How about milk and a cookie? Okay, I'll give it a try. I pour a glass of milk and plop three cookies onto a paper plate, then shuffle into the living room. Sunlight is streaming in. There's a big patch of it in the middle of the sofa. Sit, I command myself. As I sip the milk and nibble on the cookies, I start warming up. Hmmm, feeling drowsy. Good. Go with it. Pretty soon, I nod off.

The harsh ring of the phone jolts me awake. It's 10 A.M.

"Donna, I just heard the news about Eve. How is she? How are you?"

It's Jennifer, the local realtor who sold us our house. I give her a brief play-by-play, eliminating my conversation with Dr. Dave. I'm vaguely aware that I sound slightly incoherent and I'm slurring my words. I can't make my tongue cooperate.

That's confirmed by Jennifer, who says, "You don't sound very well. I'm coming over immediately. Is that okay?"

"I'm a mess, Jennifer. I need a shower. Can't stop shaking. I don't look so good."

"I don't care, if you don't care," she responds.

Actually, I'm embarrassed. But I've finally learned in life to swallow my pride in order to get help. I need help now. I need a human's touch. And Jennifer is one of the most genuinely warm people I've ever met.

"Please come," I say.

Shortly, there's a knock at the door. But before I can answer it, Jennifer lets herself in. Her aura brightens the room with her personal joie de vivre. She hurries to hug me. A look of concern clouds her sparkling eyes.

"I think I'll make us both a cup of tea," she says. "You sit down; I'll find the cups."

Jennifer wants to hear the whole story again. I oblige, this time including my conversation from last night. Her reaction is similar to Cass's. "And this cousin of Eve's is a doctor?" she asks. "Couldn't he tell you were sick? Was he trying to make you nuts?"

"No, Jennifer. I don't know him well enough for him not to like me. I think he was reeling from his conversation with the neurosurgeon. Who knows?"

"Still . . ." Jennifer shakes her head thoughtfully.

We're quiet for a while as both of us absentmindedly gaze out the window at the shimmering lake. I may have touched a nerve with Jennifer. Though ten years younger than I, she had endured more than her share of suffering. Her first son was born with the umbilical cord wrapped around his neck. He was so severely brain-damaged that he could barely breathe on his own. His lungs required suctioning all day long. Jennifer nursed him until his death in his teens.

"Nursed" might be the wrong word; "fought for him" is better. She stormed the public school system, demanding his inclusion in special education programs. I know I won't be indulging in self-pity around her.

She speaks up. "Listen, sweetie, I better go into work. Would you like to come to my house for dinner?"

"No, thanks. It's kind of you to offer. But I just can't eat these days."

"Tell you what," she says, "I'm going to ask the boss at my other job for a day off tomorrow. I'll be here at ten to take you to Green Bay to see Eve. How's that?"

I gratefully accept.

"Now, before I go, I'd like to say a prayer. Will you join me?" she asks, as she takes my hand. Truly, I am all prayed out, but I nod a half-hearted yes.

She leads. "Dear Jesus, we trust in you with all our hearts and now we come before you. You have said, 'You do not have because you do not ask.' And you told us, 'Seek and you shall find, knock and the door will be opened, ask and it will be given to you.' Dear sweet Jesus, we are asking you now for Eve's 100-percent recovery. Thank you. Amen."

Anger flushes my face. Hasn't this woman been listening to me? Eve's a vegetable. The damage is done. There's no recovery to pray for. But as quickly as the anger comes, it goes. Suddenly, an unbelievable calm descends on me, envelops me, and then fills my soul. I stop shaking. I'm awed. What's going on?

Oblivious to my range of reactions, Jennifer rises from her chair. As she reaches to hug me, a thought pops into my mind. Why not believe in Eve's 100-percent recovery? Who am I to say? Anyway, I'll go crazy thinking the other way. I open my arms to hug Jennifer.

Jennifer departs and the house is quiet once again. Too quiet. Better not sit down. Well, pacing is too much exercise. Guess I'll bite the bullet and call my A.A. sponsor. Haven't talked to her in a couple of days.

"Hi, Yolanda. How are you? Yeah, well, a lot has happened in the last 12 hours." I tell her everything. When I'm done, she punctuates the silence with an audible sigh and then asks the obvious question.

"Why didn't you call me last night?"

"Well, it was really late. I know you haven't been sleeping well with your bad back and, uh . . ."

"Excuse me," she says, "how many years have you been in this program, Donna? Since when do you decide for me whether or not I should answer a 12-Step call for help in the middle of the night?"

"Uh . . ." She has a point.

"I can't very well help you after you've lost your mind. Now listen to me. It's time to start being tough with yourself, or else you'll end up in the loony bin. Do you want to cop out like that, or are you going to face this situation and work the program on it?"

"Uh, I can try," I say. Man, is she crabby.

"So, Donna, did you read your daily meditation books this morning?"

"Not yet. But Jennifer's prayer should count for something, right?"

"Don't confuse the issue here," she says. "Jennifer's prayer is fine. But we both know you have to pray for acceptance of your role in the situation. Whether Eve recovers or not has nothing to do with how you handle today."

"But . . ." Uh-oh, I know better than to utter a "but" to my sponsor. "I mean, you're right. My priority is getting through the day. Okay, what should I do next?"

"Gather together all of your daily meditation books. Look in their indexes for the pages on 'acceptance' and read every one until you fall asleep. Then call me back when you wake up . . . refreshed and, perhaps, a little more sane and serene."

"But . . ." Damn, I did it again.

"No buts about it. You know that word H-A-L-T. We can't let ourselves get too hungry, angry, lonely, or tired. Your job is to do the next right thing. Sleep," she commands. "Everything else is out of your control," she continues. "You are powerless over Eve's coma and your financial situation. So let go and let God figure it out."

"I don't think I can do this, Yo. I can't take care of a vegetable for the rest of my life." I'm whimpering; tears are filling my eyes.

"Are you taking care of a vegetable today? How do you know what God's plan is for you? Your life is none of your business."

"But . . ." Oh, screw it.

"What have you learned from this program? In life, we sometimes have to do the things we don't want to do. Maybe this time you'll learn that lesson, gut level. There is absolutely no doubt in my mind that, if the situation were reversed, Eve would be there for you. Think about that. Then read, go to sleep, and call me. I'll be here for you, just like I would have been last night if you had picked up that phone. Good-bye. Oh, and I love you, babe."

Yes, I guess she does. I hang up and begin the process of surrender to the reality of my life and my powerlessness over the path it's taking today.

# 7

# Farewell and Good Luck

Friday morning, I am a little perturbed at how nervous I am as I dress for my first hospital visit in four days. I feel like a bad little girl for not having been there and done my duty. Lord knows I've called the nurses' station morning, noon, and night to check on Eve. But no matter which nurse I talk to, it's always the same report.

"No change," a flat voice responds, then silence. It makes no difference whether I sound cheerful or concerned, the conversation dies and I'm forced to hang up the phone. Afterward, I just want to scream, but the cats are never around when I need them.

As I watch Jennifer drive up, I warn myself not to secretly harbor any expectations for Eve's recovery. Unmet expectations will send me spiraling into self-pity. I cannot afford to go down again.

It's a good thing I talked to myself because, truly, there is no change in Eve's condition. She's still dead to the world. And so it goes. Saturday, Sunday, Monday, Tuesday, Wednesday. I keep missing the surgeon on his rounds, but he leaves me messages with the nurses. All are variations on the "nothing we can do but wait" theme.

Thursday morning, I arrive at the hospital earlier than usual for me. I want to see Eve before her two childhood friends, Liza and Karen, arrive from Chicago for a two-day visit.

As always, I take a deep breath before I enter Eve's ICU room. Then I bounce in with a cheerful "How are you doing, Eve? It's me, Donna." As I bend down to kiss her, Eve's eyelids flutter open. She recognizes me and smiles. I'm stunned. I babble, "It's me. It's you." Before I can call for a nurse, Eve's face twitches and she's gone again.

Am I nuts? Did I see what I saw? I back out of the room; one eye's on Eve, hoping it will happen again, the other eye is frantically searching for a nurse. Finally, I grab the attention of Eve's assigned nurse. Like a woman possessed, I spew out every detail of the 15-second miracle I just witnessed.

I notice the nurse is looking at me like I'm not all there, an expression of impatient "patience" written all over her face. When I'm done spewing, she responds in that too-familiar flat tone. "Yes, Eve's been doing that for a couple of hours. We have a call in to the neurologist. You saw her twitch. That's a vasospasm. You know, like a little brain seizure. Try not to stimulate her, please." The nurse whirls around and walks away.

If she had punched me in the stomach, it couldn't have hurt more. I can't bring myself to go in to see Eve. Instead, I walk out of ICU and proceed to the blissfully quiet waiting room. I've just got to hold it together for another couple of hours until Eve's friends arrive. Then I can run home—far away from this place—and stare at my lake for the rest of the day.

Liza and Karen finally arrive. Thankfully, I get involved in cushioning the blow of Eve's appearance to first-time visitors. The nurses willingly allow Eve's friends in. They even joke with them about Chicago. So, what am I, chopped liver? No, I tell myself. You're the reason Eve is in this state, and the nurses all know it and won't let you forget it. At least, that's how it feels to me.

We walk into Eve's room together. Karen and Liza are visibly shaken by the pallor of Eve's face. But they recover quickly. With more energy than I could muster today, they launch into a social banter, taking turns playing Eve's "role" in their usual three-way conversations. As if on cue, Eve's eyes open again. She smiles and makes a noise, twitches, and goes out again. Karen and Liza can barely contain their ecstasy. I want to cry.

I start to explain about overstimulation and the vasospasms, but then I shut up. Why should I put a damper on their enthusiasm? Let the nurses explain. Who knows? Maybe the two of them can make a psychic connection with Eve. A spontaneous healing? What difference does it make? Let the three of them enjoy each other's company their way. I say my good-byes . . . and tell Eve I'll see her on Saturday. As I open the door to leave, a nurse walks past me and begins chatting with them. Yeah, let her tell them.

On my way out, I run into the neurologist. He explains that the vasospasms, which are constrictions of the blood vessels, typically occur the second week after brain surgery. Luckily, Eve has not experienced any major seizures. If the vasospasms continue at this rate for another day, however, he will be forced to medicate her. Otherwise, Eve will fry her brain.

I know how stupefying seizure control medicine is. If Eve is sedated, then how will she ever come out of the coma, I ask.

The doctor just shakes his head. "We must control the spasms," he says.

Surprisingly, Friday evening, I speak with a positively chatty ICU nurse on the phone. Earlier in the day, Eve had seemed to respond to her friends' singing of Polish songs from their childhood. But then the doctor had ordered the start-up of the seizure control medicine. Eve is now resting comfortably and, predictably, unresponsive to the nurse's attempts to stimulate her.

For the next week, I continue my hospital pilgrimages and night-time calls to ICU. If it's possible for a person to look deader than dead, that's Eve. On Saturday night, before I can call ICU, the nurses call me. In that forever-flat tone, the nurse announces that they are in the process of moving Eve to intermediate ICU.

"That's good news, isn't it?" I ask optimistically. "I was just there today. Did Eve come out of the coma this evening?"

"No, there is no change," the nurse replies emphatically. "We need the ICU bed for someone else. Be sure to ask reception for the new room number. Also, your social services caseworker wants you to stop by her office on Monday." Luckily, we're not in the same room because I want to punch the living daylights out of her.

Coincidentally, earlier today, Cass had unraveled the mystery of the nurses' cold, unfeeling treatment of me. "They are 'hanging the crepe,'" Cass had announced, obviously proud of her sleuthing and acquisition of this bit of hospital jargon.

"Who told you that?" I asked.

"This friend of mine who is an ER nurse. I ran into her while grocery shopping. I asked her why in the world these nurses were acting this way toward you, since neither one of us ever experienced anything like that with hospital nurses."

"You can say that again," I reply. "But what does it mean? I don't get it."

"Oh, you know, 'hanging the crepe,' like a funeral parlor. The nurses don't want you to have any false hopes that Eve is going to come out of this."

"Hey, Cass, thanks for the insight," I say, my words dripping with sarcasm. Is she nuts? Oh, well, she must have had a tough day at work or something. Or maybe the whole world has gone mad.

The next day, Sunday, Eve's cousin Dr. Dave and his wife, Tricia, keep their promise to visit Eve. I've noticed over the past week that Eve's level of unconsciousness seems to vary. A couple of times Eve has actually half-opened her eyes, allowing me to pretend she's responding to my presence. Today is one of those good days.

Burly, outgoing, and intense, Dr. Dave announces his presence in the doorway of Eve's room. Unlike the gruff, impersonal terrorizer of my soul that I talked to two weeks ago, Dr. Dave has reverted to the charming teddy-bear man I remember meeting several years before.

"Hey, kiddo," he says to the unconscious Eve in a warm baritone voice, "how's my little pal doing?" He turns to me. "And how are you doing, Donna? Are you taking care of yourself?"

"I'm doing better," I say. "The bronchitis is finally gone. Say, Tricia, what's that?"

"Oh, I know how the nurses love to nibble. Thought I'd bring them a platter of dried fruit and nuts." She adds cheerily, "We want to keep them happy, don't we?"

Over my dead body, I say to myself.

Dr. Dave is sitting on the bed with Eve. He calls out, "Say, Donna, hand me a couple of those mouth swabs. Tricia, give me that bottle of fruit juice you've been sipping on. We're going to give Eve's taste buds a little excitement. Here, Eve, let's clean your mouth up first. Open wide. That-a-girl."

Even though Eve's eyes are still closed, I can feel an energy change in the room. Big Dr. Dave is a natural healer. I know Eve's responding to that voice.

I watch as Dr. Dave plunges a swab into the fruit juice, then coaxes Eve to open her mouth and suck on her taste treat. Over and over he does it, one swab at a time, until the bottle is empty. "There you go, Eve," he kisses her cheek. "Wasn't that fun?"

I swear Eve nods yes.

He turns to me. "Don't you go trying that," he cautions. "Do it wrong and she can aspirate it. Okay?"

He stands up. "Well, come on, Donna. Let's see what the cafeteria has for lunch. Our treat. Then we have to take off. See how close to home we can get tonight."

Throughout the week, Eve continues her comatose state. That's what I call it, but the medical profession prefers the term "level of consciousness." On that rating scale, Eve is mostly "2L," meaning she is "lethargic" and responds to loud voices and prodding. To me, that sounds relatively hopeful.

So when I meet with the caseworker and neurologist that week,

I am rather surprised by the "real" prognosis. During the meeting, I learn that the hospital is very concerned about Eve's insurance coverage. Coma or not, Eve will be discharged from the hospital in a week. If she is not out, I will be personally responsible for the hospital bill. The insurance company has spoken.

No, they say, I cannot take her home; it will be impossible for me to care for her 24/7.

According to the caseworker, they will arrange a meeting with Social Services in Green Bay. (Eve is now technically a resident of Brown County.) Social Services will show me how to "qualify" Eve for financial aid so that a nursing home will accept her. Left unsaid is that no nursing home in its right mind would take a comatose patient with only 12 days of extended care coverage, without a guarantee of state/federal aid.

Just in case I don't understand the need for a nursing home, the neurologist makes his point. Eve's brain waves are triphasic, which, as best as I understand, means that nothing is working right on a conscious level. The "good" news is that her metabolic functions are pretty normal. This fact alone makes the doctors think twice about actually calling her a "vegetable."

In other words, since Eve can breathe, poop, and pee, all is not lost? Okay, we'll continue to ride the merry-go-round of professional care.

I dutifully keep my appointment with Social Services. There, I officially learn the answer to my burning question. Yes, Eve can keep the house. But, after reducing her assets to $2,000, there's no way she can maintain it. And, since she's virtually a vegetable, she wouldn't know how to maintain it. I do. Although I could put my share of the money into maintenance, I have no legal claim to this house.

After the meeting—and time-outs for my tears—the social worker escorts me into the hall. There she suggests—off the record—that I take whatever money I am legally entitled to right now and run as far and as fast as I can.

Good idea. But for now I must play my Scarlet O'Hara role and "think about that tomorrow." Today I have an appointment with the fourth and final nursing home on my list, kindly furnished by the hospital caseworker.

By now, I'm a pro when it comes to answering the administrators' question on how Eve will pay for continuing care. "We are 'in process' on Eve's application for financial aid," I say. "Meanwhile, insurance will cover the first 12 days. Through the magic of credit cards, I will personally guarantee payment until the first of the year." This statement is always accompanied by my big confident smile. And three for three administrators have all responded with silent, disbelieving stares that naïve creatures like me actually exist and function in modern society.

The fourth nursing home would be an oddity on the Chicago scene. It is truly family-owned. Though not ritzy by any standards, I note that it's clean and free of that institutional "smell." Right off the bat, I like Faye, the admissions director, a fortyish nurse with kind eyes. Joining our meeting is the financial director who, I quickly learn, is involved in her own stroke caregiving situation with an in-law.

Based on those financial discussions with the previous three nursing homes, I've recognized that the usual balance of power has shifted. I am not interviewing them. They are determining whether Eve and I, the crazy caregiver with a credit card, are worth the financial risk.

All of the nursing home administrators have been to the hospital to evaluate Eve. Not one of them has agreed with my amateur assessment that Eve will only require a nursing home until January 1, when I have determined that she will be healthy enough to participate in an in-hospital rehabilitation program. That is, no one agreed it was remotely possible until I met Nurse Faye.

"I saw Eve yesterday," Faye says. "I believe there's a chance she could come out of this. I saw something in her eyes."

"She opened her eyes for you?" I ask incredulously. "Eve hasn't opened her eyes for me in three days. Wow! Would your nursing home's rehab staff work with Eve to get her ready for the hospital rehab?"

Faye gives me a warm smile. "We'll certainly make that one of our goals. Yes." She turns to the financial administrator. "I have a bed open. Will you approve her financially?"

"Presuming you have an excellent credit record," she nods at me, "yes, Faye, I'll approve it."

Who gets gushy about a nursing home? Me. I love the place. No, not the linoleum halls and the old-fashioned curtains, but the vibes. Even the nurse's aide, carrying a mop and pail, has a smile on her face. Though I could have chosen a closer nursing home in Door County, I am convinced that the energy and attitude of the staff will make the longer daily trip to Green Bay worth it for me and, I hope, for Eve.

# 8

# Twelve Days . . . but Who's Counting

Everything's on a roll toward Eve's discharge from the hospital Friday morning. On Wednesday, her feeding tube is scheduled to be relocated from her nose to her stomach. Usually, it's a simple outpatient procedure. Since Eve is unconscious, however, surgery and anesthesia are required, thereby guaranteeing that the costs will exceed the "usual and customary charges" the insurance company is willing to reimburse.

Predictably, Eve's friends and relatives have chosen this weekend to visit. On the one hand, I'm grateful for the support; on the other hand, I fear my social skills will fail me with so many things on my plate.

Friday morning is also the preset time for Social Security to call and interview me to see if Eve qualifies for disability. I arrange for Eve to be transported the five miles to the nursing home by medical "bus." I'm trying hard not to entertain a vision of unconscious Eve being wheeled out of the hospital and into a bus. But what else can I do? Luckily, the nursing home will postpone the admission-paper signing ceremony until I arrive in the early afternoon.

Meanwhile, Eve's sister-in-law, Arlene, and her husband, Jim, want to drive up from Chicago's O'Hare airport Wednesday, after taking an afternoon flight from Atlanta. For their own sake, I try to talk them out of their brutal travel schedule. In the end, they spend the night in Milwaukee and drive to the hospital in Green Bay on Thursday, allowing me to stay at home to clean the bathroom and reintroduce the kitchen floor to the mop.

On another front, Helen and Penny, Eve's buddies from her college days at Loyola/Rome, have also selected this weekend to visit. I can vaguely recall the size of Eve's half-room at the nursing home. I already know there will be no room for me. Oh well, I'll just sign the papers, then wait outside and smoke cigarettes until one of the visitors comes out for air.

Wednesday, Dr. Brum, the neurosurgeon, meets with me in Eve's room for a final word. I haven't seen him for several weeks; the neurologist was considered the primary physician. To Dr. Brum, I will listen. He has never given me the message that he was too "professional" to care about Eve or me.

"So, you're taking Eve to Benjamin Nursing Home," he says. "A wise decision. I had heard you wanted to bring her home."

"Not wanted to, doctor; forced to. Eve has only 12 days of nursing home insurance coverage. After that, I'll private-pay to the end of the year. Then, if she doesn't qualify for inpatient rehabilitation, I'll have no choice but to bring her home, as far as I can see."

He shakes his head. "Oh, no, you can't possibly handle Eve by yourself. You don't have family to help. Even then . . . well, it would be very difficult. The best thing you can do for Eve, and yourself, is to put her in a nursing home for a year—and then see what you've got."

"Perhaps you're right, doctor. But then I will have to give up what I've put into our house, because we'll lose it to the bank in order for me to pay a nursing home. So I'll have to figure out a different way, won't I? Maybe God will let her come out of the coma, and then she can go to a rehab hospital, covered by insurance."

"You understand that Eve has to maintain consciousness—stay alert—for three consecutive hours to participate in the rehab program here."

"Oh, I know," I agree. "Three minutes would be a miracle right now. I intend to pray a lot."

He shakes his head, then shakes my hand, and reminds me we have an appointment in a month for Eve's checkup.

I finish packing Eve's stuffed animals, including Carmel the cat, a gift from Liza, beloved by Eve and a couple of the nurses. One nurse actually gave Carmel a bath after she accidentally sprayed it with medicine. Almost done. Oh, can't forget mouth swabs. I grab two handfuls. Is this stealing? Nah, I'm sure the cost will be covered by whatever monumental bill I receive for nearly a month of ICU-level care and three surgeries.

That evening, as I'm planning my housecleaning routine for Thursday, I realize that I'm looking forward to houseguests again. We (the cats and I) have been lonely. Ozzie seems to be taking it particularly hard. He used to sleep at the foot of Eve's bed. But ever since the aneurysm, he's avoided that position like the plague. Instead, he's taken to laying his 20 pounds of cat fat on my feet every night. Maybe he'll prefer the guests' feet to mine.

I am anticipating Arlene and Jim's visit, primarily because they make me feel like family and, secondarily, because they know all about "brain" caregiving. Their young adult son, Jay, suffered severe traumatic brain injury in an auto accident several years ago. They rejected the long-term nursing home option and chose to care for him at home. As long as I had known Eve, I had heard stories of Arlene's relentless pursuit of cutting-edge rehabilitation methods for Jay.

An ingenious do-it-yourselfer, Jim had converted part of their house into a rehab unit. He also designed and built various mechanical assists, to enable them to care for big, strapping, Jay on the premises. They were also able to recruit volunteers from their parish church to help lighten the load. I know their circumstances are very different from mine, but I'm hoping we can brainstorm some ideas for Eve.

Arlene and Jim arrive Thursday evening safe and sound, and very tired. After a "Donna" dinner of cold cuts, cheeses, and ice cream, everyone's ready for bed. On Friday morning, I make up for last night's dinner with a delicious store-bought coffee cake.

Happily, Jennifer stops by and, voila, we've created a brain trust of experienced "brain" caregivers. As we sit around the table, consuming coffee and cake, Jim regales us with the story of how he designed and built a pulley system that helps them lift six-foot, two-inch Jay into a sitting position for bathing and other personal-care needs. As my mind races around trying to visualize a similar setup for our living room, only Jennifer notices that my eyes are getting wider and that my skin is turning green.

"Excuse me, Jim," Jennifer interrupts. "I may be out of line, but we don't have to go there yet. Donna is overwhelmed enough with the nursing home transfer. Eve will not be home for at least eight weeks. Donna doesn't have to plan home care this week."

"Oh, yeah, sorry," Jim responds.

Jennifer continues, "But I'm sure there's a lot you can tell her about dealing with Eve's coma. That's the help she needs now."

Click. Thank God, my mind stops building Rube Goldberg contraptions in the living room. I nod at Jennifer, deeply grateful for the halting of my downward slide into the muck of too much information.

And, thankfully, Arlene picks up on what Jennifer said and proceeds to tell me how she dealt with the day-to-day of Jay's coma. Soon after, Jim joins in with his experiences and reactions.

"Music," Jim says. "Bring a CD player and Eve's favorite upbeat music to the nursing home this weekend. Get her to 'dance.'"

"Treats for the nurses' aides," Arlene adds. "You want to encourage them to visit Eve when you're not there. You can't do this alone."

So it goes, until it's time for them to go to the hospital to oversee Eve's transfer, while I wait for Social Security's 11 A.M. call.

And then the call comes. The disembodied voice of Social Security speaks. "We have all of Eve's records. We understand she is disabled and the condition may be permanent. But Eve does not have enough quarters with income from earned wages to qualify for Social Security disability on her own." And the final shocker: "No, Eve does not qualify for widow's disability on her husband's Social Security because he's been dead more than seven years. Do you have anything that would refute this?"

"No, I guess not."

"We'll send you our decision in the mail. Sorry. Good-bye."

Okay, that went well. Now, I have to resist the panic-borne urge to return to bed and bury my head under the covers. "Can't go there," I say aloud. Instead, I hug the cats for a couple of minutes. Unfortunately, they just don't understand. Gotta get dressed; try to look nice for the guests and the nursing home staff. Move, I command myself.

At the nursing home, I seek out Eve's room to find Arlene. On the drive over, I decided to recruit her to sit with me through the paper-signing process. After all, if something happens to me, somebody will have to take care of Eve. And that somebody is not going to be Vivian, who never bothered calling to tell me she wasn't going to co-sign the power of attorney document.

Afterward, I return to Eve's room with Arlene. Walking down the hall, I can tell from the commotion that Penny and Helen have arrived from Chicago. You'd think it was a New Year's bash going on, with all the whooping, laughter, and high-energy conversation coming from Eve's room.

Inside, Jim is kicking Eve's bed, rousing her from the coma with pure, brute force. Helen is crying and Penny's shouting into Eve's ear as if she's deaf: "Eve, only 12 days of nursing home coverage! Do you hear me? Come out of that coma right now! You've got to be out of here in 12 days! Are you listening, Eve?"

Amazingly, Eve's eyes are open, a big smile on her face, and she's nodding to one and all. The entire scene is a madhouse!

"Hi, everyone," I say. "Thanks for coming. I need a cigarette now." Yep, I'm the first visitor to run outside and gulp the fresh air.

Before we depart the nursing home, Arlene and Jim insist that they will treat us to pizza delivery tonight. I can understand their desperation for real food; unfortunately, those big-city conveniences aren't available mid-November in a tourist town. Instead, I suggest they join Penny and Helen for dinner in Green Bay. I'll head on home. I need some time alone to feel sorry for myself.

On Saturday, I have plenty of time to do just that. Jim and Arlene head back to Chicago after breakfast. They promise to stop at the nursing home on their way. Helen and Penny, who spent the night in a Green Bay motel, will see Eve around noon and then head back. Meanwhile, I can rest up for my first solo visit tomorrow.

Sunday morning, 10 A.M. I'm all set to embark for Green Bay when the thought occurs, "Gee, I'll be traveling to Green Bay at the same time as thousands of fanatical Packer football fans, many of whom spent the night in Door County." That would be very dumb. I decide to wait an hour and . . . what else? Occupy my mind by thinking too much.

Finally on my way to Green Bay, I amuse myself by flipping between the Packers and the Bears on the car radio. In those pre-aneurysm days, Eve and I would be doing just that with the TV remote control on any given autumn Sunday. I make a mental note to dispense with the costly package required to receive Chicago Bears football via satellite on TV. I won't need that for a while.

At the nursing home, I walk through the TV lounge en route to Eve's room. All the ambulatory residents and some of the staff are gathered around the tube, cheering on their Green Bay gods. It's my first real taste of this town's mania for their beloved Packers. Kind of seems like fun. But that's not on the agenda today, so I keep walking down the hall to Eve's room.

Poor kid, she's dead to the world again. She's pooped from all the excitement. It's my first opportunity to meet Eve's roommate, a sweet elderly lady who has obviously suffered a stroke. Her words are slightly garbled, but eventually I understand what she's saying. Yes, Eve is very pretty. Yes, I know the nurses can't wake her up, no matter how hard they try. You're right; she is too young to be here. Yeah, it is a shame, a damned shame.

# Twelve Days . . . but Who's Counting

I sit down in the recliner next to Eve's bed. The muted TV in the room is tuned to—guess what—the Packers' game. An hour passes. Home team's winning; Eve's still sleeping. Finally, it's over—the game and my visit. I don't want to drive at dusk. That's when the deer come out to play chicken with the cars. Eve has not budged since my arrival. I kiss her good-bye and leave.

On the way home, I review my new reality in my head. "Be sure to bring a book," Cass had suggested during her regular nightly phone call to me. A good idea, but lately, I can't even concentrate on a tabloid story, let alone a novel. I better figure out some way to pass the time or I'll bore myself to death on these visits.

I've been lost in thought for a while when I notice I'm passing the third country tavern in ten minutes. The parking lots are jammed with cars of fans celebrating the Packers victory. Before I know it, I'm imagining the good time everyone is having inside the bar. Gosh, I'm thirsty. Wouldn't a frosty beer taste good now? All of a sudden I realize how desperately I want to stop at the next tavern and join them.

"God, no. Please don't let me drink."

I want a beer so bad. No, I don't. Yes, I do. No, Donna, what you want so badly is oblivion. You just don't care anymore. But Cass will kill you if she hears you slurring your words when she calls tonight.

That's easy; I just won't answer the phone. For the next three days? Have you forgotten your last drinking days? You won't stop until they cart you off. Remember, Yolanda said your next stop would be a mental ward, not some fancy-shmantsy treatment center.

Okay, yeah. I'm breaking into a sweat. Finding it hard to focus. "Drive, Betsy," I command the car. "Take me home, country road." It's okay if you leave town tonight, but you can't drink today. Now, go home and pack, if you want to run away. But you'll run sober. Now pray and drive.

Finally, I hear the driveway gravel crunching under my tires. Quickly, I park the car and run around the house to the lakeside. Breathing deeply, I beg the infinite blue for help. "Please." It's the only prayer I can pray. "Please, help me." Okay, I'm calming down.

H-A-L-T, I remind myself. You're hungry, tired, lonely, too. Go inside, eat, and call somebody.

Inside, I'm greeted by two cats and a blinking answering machine. It's Jennifer, offering to accompany me to the nursing home on Tuesday. I call back. Surely, she won't be home on this beautiful Sunday afternoon.

"Hello," Jennifer answers. So much for my ESP. We chat a bit about the visitors and set the time for Tuesday. The conversation is winding down. I'd better take advantage of the break God has given me.

"Say, Jennifer, remember I told you I'm in A.A.? Well, if you have a second, I think I better describe my trip home today. It will help if I come clean. No, I didn't drink, but I came awfully close." I tell her about my battle with myself.

"Do I want to drink now? No, not at this moment, thanks to your call. But I know my sponsor's out of town and Cass won't be calling until late; she's at a wedding, I believe. Oh, sure, thanks. Yes, I'm getting a pencil right now. Yes, I'm writing down the number. Yes, I will. Thanks. See you Tuesday."

Oh, rats. Just my luck that Jennifer's good friend Adrienne is in A.A. in Door County. I promised to call her, and Jennifer's going to know if I don't. Darn. Well, guess I'll call her now. Maybe she's out on this lovely afternoon and I can get away with leaving a message.

I dial, and guess what? She's home, too. Not only is she home, but she offers to meet me at the 7:00 A.A. meeting in Egg Harbor. Damn. Rats. Sure, I will. I hang up. Now I'm really hungry.

It's not that I don't believe an A.A. meeting could help me, but I've been rationalizing for several weeks how the phone calls back to my Chicago A.A. roots were enough to get me through this crisis. Truth is, Eve and I were pretty sloppy about going to meetings regularly our first year here. It's not always comfortable, breaking into a new group. We excused ourselves from A.A. by saying we'd get back into the routine after our house was rehabbed.

"You're taking an A.A. vacation," my sponsor would warn. "Dipping into that A.A. bank account. Hope your serenity holds out until you find the time to do what you're supposed to do."

I guess time's up.

I'm back from the meeting by 8:20. Yes, I promised Adrienne I'd meet her again Friday night. And I will give her a call during the week. But my A.A. adrenalin is pumping now. Who can I call?

Why, Ginny, of course. God love her. She was our closest A.A. pal in Sedona, Arizona. I haven't called to tell her about Eve's aneurysm. Didn't want to upset her. After all, she's 90-something now. Uh, who are you kidding, Donna? Ginny also has 50-plus years of sobriety. She's an A.A. pioneer. Even knew Bill Wilson, our founder, well enough to say hi. Naw, you won't shock Ginny.

"Hi there, kiddo," Ginny's raspy voice greets me as she recognizes mine. "How's tricks?"

I offer her the condensed version of Eve's aneurysm story. Don't want to tire her before I get to the meat of the conversation.

"So what are you going to do while Eve's in a coma?" she asks.

"Pray for acceptance," I answer in true A.A. fashion.

"Oh, horsefeathers," she scoffs at me. "Sounds to me like you've set up some mighty high expectations for Eve's recovery. Didn't you just say you hoped she'd be ready for rehab by January first? Or is my hearing aid turned off?"

Oh, pigeon poop. She's on to me.

"Remember what I always say?" she asks. "No matter how hard one beats at the portals of night, daylight will come at the appointed time. Well, do you remember that?"

"Yes, ma'm," I say. "Thank you, I do. But I don't like it."

"Who gives a fiddle what you like? Like it or not, you better start dealing with life on life's terms. You know I can't stand whiney women. Buck up."

"This brings me to one more thing, Ginny. This afternoon." I'm trying hard not to sound meek, but my wimpiness is leaking out. I tell her about my close encounter with the bars. After I finish, there is a very long, dramatic pause. "Ginny, are you there?" I ask, hoping we've been disconnected.

"Oh, I'm here, dearie. But I'm just appalled by what I'm hearing from my little protégé. I thought I had taught you something while you were here. I presume you realize that if the circumstances were the other way around, Eve would take care of you."

I really wish I didn't have to be told this twice, but I guess God thinks I'm deaf. "Yes, Ginny, I have no doubt."

"Then I don't ever want to hear you whimper again about how close you came to picking up a drink. You are going to handle this crisis with dignity. Do you understand?"

Oh, boy, do I? I'm turning red with shame. Ginny has hit a nerve.

"I can't stand whining," she adds, as if she needs to.

"I understand. No more."

"Now, that's my girl. I'm getting a little tired now. You'll call and let me know what happens, please." I realize that I haven't asked her how she's doing. Man, I'm batting a thousand today. But I can hear that she's tired now. Another time.

"Okay, thanks, Ginny. Please take care of yourself."

# 9

# Go, Lions

It doesn't matter how I look at it, it's difficult to motivate myself for a daily three-hour round-trip to visit with comatose Eve on these bleak November days. This might be easier if I could see a light at the end of the tunnel. But, honestly, I can't say that I do.

Arlene and Cass have tried their best at "cheerleading" by suggesting I talk to Eve about our dreams. They believe, as I do, that people in comas can hear and that my words will register at some level. If only I had dreams to communicate. Eve and I didn't really share a "happily ever after" vision. Neither of us wanted to travel around the world nor to retire anywhere but to our little lakefront house. Fame and fortune held no allure; we were just grateful to have escaped alive from our personal battles with alcoholism.

In reality, we were content to lead a relatively quiet life, spiced up with weekend TV football games, art gallery tours, and, perhaps, an annual trip to Las Vegas to dump our excess savings. None of it was coma-breaking dream material.

Truth be told, I wasn't confident that Eve wanted to hear the sound of my voice. I couldn't shake the feeling that Eve was resisting my suggestions to "come to," because she knew what I was going to say about our finances. They were a mess, despite her insistence that everything was under control. At some level, I believe Eve realized that once I got past the joy of her coming out of the coma, I'd be harping on her to get busy and help me figure out how to promote my artwork or a gallery. That was W-O-R-K. Work was, and still is, a four-letter word to Eve. She had been lucky enough to have escaped the need for it most of her life. Who would want to "wake up" to find out her world has changed and reality is biting her behind?

However, I am the only person around who has a shot at enticing her back into reality. Obviously, this will work better if I can maintain a cheerful and enthusiastic presence at her bedside. For this reason alone, it behooves me to come up with a strategy to motivate myself to make my visits meaningful, at least, and fun, at most.

So for the first few days I work on setting up a reasonable visitation schedule. With no audience of friends or relatives to play to, the idea of being a martyr who shows up every day without fail is not alluring. Right now, Eve is receiving some stimulation from physical and speech therapy during the week. I want her minimally stimulated every day. That makes my weekend visiting imperative.

I decide that Wednesdays and Thursdays will be my days off— one day for housework, one for paying bills. I set my schedule for 10 A.M. to 2 P.M., so I don't interfere with her personal-care routine and I don't have to drive in fear of deer at dusk.

In between, I can monitor whatever therapy is scheduled, plus wait for the "magic" moments. Yes, it's my new game. While I sit next to Eve, I make sporadic attempts at one-way communication, but mostly I lie in wait for the moment she coughs, changes foot position, or otherwise appears restless. Then I go for it.

"Eve, wake up. Come on, Eve, it's Donna. I can only visit for a short time, so I need you to open your eyes now. Come on, Eve, give me a smile. Talk to me; I'm bored. That-a-girl, look at me, Eve. Say something. Wake up. Here, I'll give you a reward. I will clean your mouth with a swab, if you'll just wake up for a moment. Please."

I might get such an opportunity four or five times during my daily visit. I consider the day a success if she "comes to" for ten or 15 seconds, just once. More days than not, I "win."

One day, as we're approaching Eve's two-week nursing home anniversary, Faye, the nurse, stops to visit us. "I was hoping you'd be here," she says. "I want to talk to you."

"Isn't that coincidental," I respond, "because I was just about to go looking for you. I have been wondering about something."

"What's on your mind?" Faye asks.

"I know I shouldn't play doctor; but I've been thinking about Eve's medications. I am going to talk about my experience first. I've been on one antidepressant after another since the day Prozac was invented. Every time I start a new one, the doctor prescribes some huge dosage to begin. I always end up complaining about being 'dopey' after a week and begging the doctor for a decrease in dosage.

"Anyway, it seems to me that Eve is on an awfully high dose of seizure-control medicine. Look at how tiny she is. Do you think that part of this coma might be due to her being overmedicated?"

"That's so weird," Faye says, "because that's why I wanted to talk to you. It's my feeling, too."

"So how are we going to approach the neurologist on that one? Last time we spoke," I say, "he was still concerned about Eve's seizures."

"Well," Faye responds, "she hasn't had any seizures here. But don't worry, I'll talk to him and let you know what he says. We can only try."

Two days later, after my midweek home maintenance holiday, I return to the nursing home for my Friday visit. One of the nurses waves at me as I walk in. "Hey, Donna," she says, "Faye said to tell you that the medicine reduction has begun. Also, she said not to expect any change right away. Give it a week."

Of course, I expect a change right away. But when I walk into Eve's room, she's not dancing on the TV. As usual, she's "comatosing."

However, that day she "comes to" twice during those "magic" moments. I hardly dare to hope.

Over the weekend, I try not to impose my will on what I see happening with Eve. But gosh, it sure seems like she's at a higher level of consciousness. Ah, heck, what do I know?

Now it's Thanksgiving week, so I decide to take off Tuesday and Wednesday. I fear Thanksgiving will be a little brutal emotionally. Though the nursing home tries to make the holiday festive for the residents, Eve is unconscious and on a feeding tube. No turkey for her . . . or me.

On Thanksgiving Eve, I'm immersed in paying a pile of bills when the phone rings at 6 P.M. It's Marie calling. She's a nurse who primarily handles staffing at the nursing home. But since Eve is the only "private pay" resident in the home, it appears that poor Marie also got "stuck" with the job of acting as liaison with the insurance company. On various occasions, Marie has told me that she admires my gutsy request that their staff should "stand by for rehabilitation" when Eve comes out of the coma.

Marie begins, "Are you sitting down, Donna?"

"Yeah, what's wrong, Marie? Geez, I knew I should have gone in today."

"Nothing's wrong. Take it easy. This is good news."

"Good news? What's that?"

"Let me tell you how I championed Eve's cause." I can almost hear her puffing up. "I've become quite chummy with Eve's insurance caseworker over the phone in the past week or so." Puff. Puff.

I do like this girl. "That's good to hear, Marie. I've never talked to the insurance caseworker. Everybody tells me to let you experts handle it."

"Well, I have been handling it," Marie continues. "It's currently my favorite challenge. So guess what? I just got off the phone with insurance. They have agreed to take this calendar year's inpatient hospital rehabilitation and apply it toward the nursing home because, as I explained to them, Eve's receiving excellent therapy here."

"Oh, my God." It's all I can say.

"Now I'll have to report to them on a week-to-week basis. And Eve will have to improve. But you are potentially covered by insurance until Christmas. How's that for a Thanksgiving present?"

"I want to kiss you, Marie. Buy you chocolates . . . flowers . . . anything you want. Thank you for caring, for trying. And . . . oh man, just thank you."

Eventually, I run out of breath and we hang up. Finally, I have some good news to share with the people who really care. In the middle of my telephone marathon, I receive a call from our next-door neighbors, a retired couple, Norm and Doris. They have called several times in the past few weeks to invite me to dinner. I've begged off on these occasions, primarily because of my lack of appetite . . . and, well, I felt awkward.

Prior to Eve's aneurysm, most of our neighborly interaction was friendly but reserved, in-the-garden chats. Now they are insisting that I join them for Thanksgiving dinner. The timing is such that I have to beg off again.

"Oh, no, you don't," Doris protests. "We are saving you some turkey. Now I know you'll be tired. And maybe you won't feel like talking. But you call us when you get home tomorrow. Norm and I will bring dinner over to you. And there's absolutely no way you can get out of that. Understand?"

"Oh, jeez, you guys are just too nice. Yes, I promise I'll call. Thank you for understanding."

"You bet," Doris says. "By the way, we will expect you for dinner on Sunday, even if you can only eat dessert. I believe you once said that you like good vanilla ice cream as much as Norm does."

"Yes," I say. "I surrender. I accept. I'll be there." Thus begins my new friendship with the neighbors.

Thanksgiving morning, I arrive at the nursing home in time for the tail end of Macy's parade, but with plenty of time to chat at the desk with an excited nurse's aide.

"Eve was awake," she says, "alert through most of her morning shower. She's sort of sleeping now, but I put her in a wheelchair. Take her for a spin around the nursing home; see if she wakes up for you."

# Brain, Heal Thyself

Sure enough, Eve is "dozing" in the chair when I walk in. But it doesn't take all that long for me to wake her up. "Come on, Eve, we're going to explore the hallways. How's that?" Eve nods. Her eyes actually look bright. I wheel her out and we're off.

After about three minutes, Eve is sliding down in the seat, falling asleep. I stop and talk her into waking up again. "Just one more hall. Two minutes. Let's see if you can stay awake." We turn down a hall I haven't traveled before. At the end is a little room, painted bright yellow and springtime green. It's obviously a lounge, but nobody's around. There are a few garden-style chairs and a TV in the corner.

I say to Eve, "Hey, let's see how the annual Detroit Lions game is going. You know . . . football. Watching it on TV is our favorite pastime."

I'm not sure if Eve is nodding in agreement or falling asleep, but I'm on a roll. I flip on the TV and begin a play-by-play commentary on top of the announcers' chitchat. If I continue talking, maybe I can keep her in this world a little longer.

"There you go, Eve. The Lions are driving. They are such losers this year. But, hey, maybe they'll score now, make it a game. Look, there's a pass. Catch it, catch it. What? Offensive pass interference? Baloney. Did you see that?" I turn to her. "What the heck was that all about?"

I can't believe what happens next. Eve shrugs her shoulders, looks heavenward, then shakes her head. My God, she comprehends the game! She watched the TV, she saw the play, and she understood the game. It's a miracle!

I can hardly contain my glee. But there's no one around to tell. I wheel Eve back to the room and find a nurse's aide to help me put Eve to bed. She's very sleepy. I pop an easy-listening CD into the player and then kiss her good-bye, with a promise to see her tomorrow.

I fly back home. As I open the door, the phone is ringing and the cats are meowing. What joyful noise. It's Doris on the phone. She saw me drive up. She and Norm are on their way to deliver dinner. No, I can't pick it up. Then they're at the back door, each bearing a tower of plastic containers.

"We won't stay," she promises.

76

"But I want you to hear what happened," I counter. All of a sudden I've found my social skills. "Please, let me share this."

Doris claps her hands when I'm finished. "See, it works," she says to Norm. "We have three different prayer groups in Door County praying for you and Eve."

"Well, isn't that super," I say. "Add to that two in Evanston, one in Naperville, and one in Kentucky. I think we've got every faith covered, too. I don't know if you've ever been on the receiving end, Doris, but I sure felt the power of prayer today. Of course, it's easy to feel it when you witness a miracle. I guess I gotta thank those groups for keeping me glued together while I was waiting for something, anything, to happen. Now that takes power."

"Amen," says Norm, as he gives me a hug. "Enjoy dinner. Doris tells me we'll be seeing you on Sunday."

"You bet. I can't thank you enough. Be careful walking back, please. It's pitch black out there."

I'm starving. I devour the eight-course carry-out dinner like I haven't had a meal in a month, which is partly true. Eve is back, and so is my appetite. The tryptophan in the turkey sends me to bed early. But then, I haven't slept very well in a while either. This time, it's straight through until morning. Oh, what a happy Thanksgiving.

I can hardly wait to get to the nursing home on Friday morning to share the good news with the physical therapy team. When I enter Eve's room, the team of Pattie and Bruce is already at work, helping Eve relearn how to sit up in bed.

"8, 9, 10 . . ." Pattie counts the stopwatch ticks. "And, whoops, there she goes, Bruce, catch her." Eve safely plops sideways on her pillow.

Pattie turns to me. "Best time yet," she declares. "We worked on her sit-up time Tuesday and Wednesday, but we missed you. Glad Eve's coming down on that medicine. We can see a big difference."

"Hey, great. What happens next?" I ask. "Do you need my help, or should I just stay out of the way?"

Bruce speaks up. "If you'll just hold that wheelchair by the door steady, that'll help. We want to bring Eve down to our therapy room for a change of scenery. She's getting sleepy. We're still a ways from keeping her awake for the three-hour period the rehab hospitals require," he says with a wink to me.

"Okay," I say, "so my goal is a little overambitious. But if anybody can do it, it's you, big Bruce." I wink back.

"Uh-huh," he says. Bruce is concentrating on securing the safety belt around Eve's waist. "Okay, Pattie, are you ready? Let's get Eve to stand and then we'll each grab her under the arm, lift, and carry her over to the wheelchair. On my count, 1-2-3."

At first, I'm more surprised by Pattie's strength than anything else. But then I see it . . . and all I can do is point and wave and utter little nonsense noises. "Uh, er, uh, um, LOOK!"

They're almost to their destination when they both look down and see what I'm blabbering about. Although four inches off the floor, Eve is swishing her feet back and forth, pointing her toes down, anxiously trying to contact the floor so she can WALK to the wheelchair. Stunned, the therapists set her down. Bruce gawks at Eve's feet in disbelief. Pattie just says, "Oh, my God. Eve wants to walk. She wants to walk."

Bruce is still gawking. Finally, he stutters, "This is awesome. Let's just get her down to the therapy room right away. I have a brilliant idea."

The three of us parade down the hall, pushing Eve in her wheelchair. We're all bouncing with anticipation over what amazing feat Eve will perform next. Inside the oversized therapy room, Bruce races to a closet and disappears for a couple of minutes. Pattie and I are busy patting Eve's head a lot and prodding her to stay awake.

Finally, Bruce emerges with what looks like an enclosed walker with wheels in front. Bruce walks over to Eve's wheelchair and squats to talk to her. "How you feeling, kid? Are you strong enough to try the walker today?" She nods. "Okay. Pattie, come over here, please. Let's do it."

They lift Eve out of the chair to a standing position, holding her while I wheel the walker up to Eve. She fits inside the little cage that will keep her from tipping left or right. Pattie grabs hold of the safety belt. Eve's hands are clutching the handlebars, and I assume the role of the pied piper.

"Come, follow me, Eve," I call out. "We're going to try to make it to the door. Let's do it to it."

For the next 90 seconds, everyone's holding their breath as Eve pushes forward, one foot, then the other. Finally, she backs me out into the hall. Eve has arrived at the doorway.

"Oh gee, ooh, wow," Bruce says as he rushes up behind Eve with the wheelchair and sits her down. Once again, he squats. "Eve, do you think you can do it just one more time, p-l-e-a-s-e? I want the whole world to see this."

Eve is visibly tired; perspiration dots her forehead. Still she nods yes.

"The whole world? Wait a second, Bruce," I say. "I do want her to look pretty for the occasion." With that I spit on my fingers, fuss with her eclectic hairdo, and twirl the erratic bangs hiding her eyes. Eve smiles and gives me a look like I'm nuts.

Meanwhile, Bruce has commandeered the intercom. "Attention, all staff and everybody else, please come to the therapy room immediately and bring any ambulatory residents with you. We have a surprise."

Bruce races over to Eve and stands her up in the walker. Then he runs to the door, peeks outside, and waves to an apparently gathering crowd.

Knowing how much Eve loved the theater, I know the drama of the moment is not lost on her. Bruce signals me and I resume my pied piper role.

"Come on, Eve," I say. "It's the doorway or bust. This is your show. Follow me."

Sweat is pouring from her brow, but somehow Eve must know that fame awaits her out there in the hall of the nursing home. Ten steps, 12 steps, 15 steps, and Eve passes through the portal. The audience erupts in thunderous applause as Eve appears, smiling from ear to ear, playing the crowd. The cheers encourage her onward, adrenaline is pushing her, but, thankfully, Pattie and Bruce run up behind and coax Eve back into the wheelchair. The queen is seated on her throne and all pay homage to Eve. What a performance!

Finally, even this great moment must end. Exhausted, Eve is falling asleep while we wheel her back to the room. Bruce and Pattie lovingly lift her out of the chair and back into bed. I tuck her in.

As Bruce backs out of the room, he bows to Eve and me. "Thank you for this day, ladies. I had almost forgotten, but this is why I became a therapist. Thank you, and good-night."

# 10

# Piece of Cake

It's the first weekend of December and Eve's room is hopping. All the nurses' aides pop in and out, hoping to be rewarded by a wakeful smile from pixie Eve. Everyone knows of my quest to keep Eve awake for three continuous hours so that she can qualify for inpatient hospital rehabilitation by the first of the year. Even her friends back in Chicago want to play the game.

Cass is sending Eve a card a day designed to elicit a laugh. Other friends are sending photos with short "remember when's?" attached. I read them all to Eve every day.

Speech therapy has begun in earnest. Christine, a young attractive therapist, demonstrates a compassion for stroke victims beyond her years. I watch as she works to calm down Eve's elderly roommate, who is frustrated because she mixes up the names of kitchen utensils. Oh, how I wish Eve were that progressed. When it's Eve's turn,

Christine includes me in the process, explaining what she's doing with Eve and why. She's a natural teacher.

A major consequence of the aneurysm is the paralysis of Eve's throat and interior mouth. She can barely move her tongue; she can't chew, swallow, or speak.

My first therapy assignment is to stick out my tongue frequently at Eve and invite her to retaliate. As an added bonus, it's a nice, safe outlet for any subsurface frustration I'm feeling on any given day. "Here, Eve, take that! Waaah!" Very cathartic.

Christine also asks Eve ten yes-no questions daily to test her comprehension. Ever-compliant Eve is a fooler. After several sessions, we realize that Eve is nodding yes out of habit. Eve has obviously learned that yes usually works to get your needs met in a nursing home environment.

Other than Eve's dubious nodding in answer to a question, I have no real communication with her. That doesn't stop me from trying, however. I've bought every mentally stimulating child's book I can find, plus pipe cleaners, crayons, coloring books, pick-up-sticks, Barrel of Monkeys, and Silly Putty.

Surprisingly, I discover that all these child learning tools are not stimulating Eve to learn. In fact, I believe they are boring her. She'd rather flip through a magazine, but I can't figure out if she's looking at pictures or actually reading the words.

I'm not the only one confused by Eve. So is her new occupational therapist (though I doubt she'd ever admit it). I'm allowed to be present during these sessions, as long as I remain a spectator. Sometimes this is easier said than done.

For this morning's exercise, Dottie, the therapist, wheels Eve up to a table. In the middle is a selection of colored pegs and a color-coded wooden block of holes.

"Eve, I want you to put the green pegs in the green holes," the OT explains. "Do you understand?"

As Eve is compliantly nodding yes to the therapist, a little voice in my head is snickering. Yeah, I see that old familiar twinkle in Eve's eyes. This is going to be interesting.

"Eve," I say, crossing the "spectator" border, "you do understand green in green, red in red, don't you?" Uh-oh, was that a nod . . . and a wink?

Eve picks up a green peg. The naïve therapist is waiting expectantly. I know better. Yep, there goes the green peg . . . into Eve's mouth, now into an ear, through her hair, on the way to her nose.

"Quit it, Eve," I shout, startling poor Dottie. "Stop goofing off. Put the damn green peg in the damn green hole, or you'll be very sorry."

At that, the peg goes directly into Eve's nose, as she defiantly turns to me.

"You brat," I yell, rising from the chair threateningly.

"Whoa," Dottie intervenes, before I can put my hands around Eve's neck. "Somebody needs a cigarette break."

"But Eve knows exactly what she's doing," I protest. "She's playing us."

"We don't know that," counters the therapist.

Yes we do, I think to myself, as I fumble in my purse for the cigarettes.

"Now, best you go outside and calm down," the therapist says to me.

"Yeah, you're right," I say, as the therapist is talking nice-nice to Eve. Oh, poop, I think, as I retreat. They've yet to design an occupational therapy program that will intrigue Eve to try. I sure hope this therapist gets the message to think outside the box.

Eventually, Dottie does catch on to Eve and offers her more interesting projects. But it comes too late; Eve has her number and OT becomes one of Eve's favorite games.

On another morning, I walk into a physical therapy session in progress. For the past 20 minutes, Eve has been practicing sitting up in bed, coming from a supine position. Pattie, the physical therapist, announces that they'll be heading back to the room now. Eve, who is sitting on the edge of the cot, shifts her position so that Pattie can help her into the wheelchair. Pattie is writing notes on her clipboard when she notices the shift.

She says, "Oh, but you'll have to wait a second. Did you forget, Eve? We have to put on your gym shoes first." Then Pattie returns to her clipboard again, not noticing what I can see from across the room. Eve looks at Pattie, shrugs, then bends down, grabs her shoe, opens up the lacing, and puts it on her foot. By now, Pattie is noticing Eve, and so is Dottie, who stops working with another patient to watch the unfolding drama.

Oblivious to all of our open mouths and disbelieving stares, Eve proceeds to lace up the shoe and tie a perfect bow. Then she puts on the other shoe the same way. Dottie looks like she's going to faint. Pattie and I exchange stunned stares.

"Are you ready now, Eve?" Pattie asks. Her question sends Dottie and me into hysterics. Holy cow!

A few days later, Eve and I travel back to the hospital for the one-month checkup. The first stop is the neurologist, Dr. "Doomsday." I recite the litany of Eve's recent accomplishments. He nods impassively and says, "Well, I knew she had a recovery in her all along. Just took time." Good thing I'm not packing a pistol at that moment.

The next stop is the neurosurgeon, Dr. Brum. "So, it appears the medicine was contributing to the drowsy state. I'll be talking to the neurologist about that," he says thoughtfully. "But, more importantly, I think it's time we insert a shunt in Eve's brain. I believe she's being held back by the hydrocephalus. That's when there's too much blood and liquid on the brain. It creates pressure that interferes with balance, slows her down. We'll schedule the surgery for the Friday before Christmas."

"Is the surgery dangerous?" I ask, obviously anxious about the prospect of three brain surgeries in three months.

"Oh, no, the surgery is not dangerous. It's a piece of cake. And here's the good news . . . I think Eve will improve ten to 50 percent. I don't know what form that improvement will take. But you will see it."

He's smiling like Santa Claus. Ho-ho! His blue eyes are twinkling in the fluorescent light. Man, he is so-o-o cute . . . and to think he's a brain surgeon, too. But, alas, he's very married, so I manage to refrain from kissing him.

# Piece of Cake

Back at the nursing home, the countdown to Christmas Day has begun. The cafeteria is bedecked with a "winter wonderland" display, designed to delight the inner child of every elderly resident. Eve's social calendar is packed with concerts . . . from singing Cub Scouts, to Sweet Adelines, a one-man band, a honky-tonk piano player, and several local church choirs. Why, even Santa himself is planning to stop by with presents for all.

I'm looking forward to the weekend before Christmas. Our Chicago friends, Roger and Merle, are coming up . . . and they promise to bring Christmas with them.

I met Roger and Merle in my first days of recovery, when I was stumbling in and out of sobriety, trying desperately to understand this simple 12-Step program. With infinite patience, the two of them tried to explain how I was complicating the process. "Just don't pick up the first drink," Roger would say . . . and then he'd say it again and again, when I'd return to A.A. meetings after another relapse.

But most important to me at the time were their invitations to join their family for every holiday occasion. I wasn't alone; dozens of people benefited from their generosity over the years. They taught me that life was not only worth living without alcohol, but that it could be fun again. And we had shared some great times together since then.

Sunday afternoon, I meet them at the nursing home. It takes Roger five trips to the car to unload all the gifts. Meanwhile, Merle is lighting up the nursing home with her dazzling smile and ebullient personality; plus she's brought homemade cookies and candy for the nurses and staff.

Inside Eve's room, Merle finds the oversized carton box she's looking for . . . and presto . . . she produces a decorated, lighted Christmas tree. Then she brings out the presents. Eve receives three adorable jogging outfits (her uniform at the nursing home). I receive an entire holiday outfit, including a decorated Christmas sweatshirt. Next come Eve's new toys: an electronic update of Mr. Potato Head, a Speak and Spell machine, picture books, and puzzles galore. And Roger adds, "We're treating you, Donna, to a night stay at the motel. You'll probably be too sleepy to drive back after dinner at Brett Favre's steakhouse." Move over, Santa. Merle and Roger have arrived in Green Bay.

Over dinner that night, Merle whispers to me, "By the way, Roger and I will be picking up your mortgage payment beginning in January. We'll take care of that until you know where you stand with Eve. We don't want you to worry about finances at this time. Don't go protesting; it's just a loan."

All of us return to the nursing home the next morning. The mailman has delivered a batch of Christmas cards for Eve. Usually, I give Eve one card at a time to open, and then read it to her looking over her shoulder. But today I am seated in front of Eve, on her bed, to make room for Merle and Roger.

As I wait for Eve to finish looking at the cover of the card, I notice the process is taking longer. Could it be my imagination, or are her eyes tracking the words? When she opens the card, she does it again. I know the card is from my cousin and her husband. Eve has met them, but doesn't know them well.

"Eve," I say, "look at the signature, please. Can you tell me who this card is from?"

Eve nods.

"Okay. Who?"

"Valerie and Dale." She mouths the names.

Hallelujah! Hallelujah! Eve can read.

Now Christmas is coming way too fast, and I'm not even counting how many shopping days are left. Eve's surgery is three days away, on Friday.

On Wednesday night, I receive a call from Penny, Eve's bubbly friend from Chicago. She delivers her message in the usual rapid-fire manner. "Hi, Donna. Now don't try to talk me out of this . . . but I've decided I'm driving up to Green Bay tomorrow . . . weather's supposed to be clear . . . good driving . . . gotta wish my little buddy a 'Merry Christmas' or . . . well, you know . . ."

Penny pauses to take a breath. Now's my chance. "Do you want to spend the night here, Penny?"

"Oh, thanks, but no." She's off and running again. "I figured if I leave at seven . . . I'll be up by noon . . . and that means I have four hours to visit with Eve . . . then I'll take you to dinner somewhere . . . you pick . . . Merry Christmas . . . then I'll head back . . . get going before it's too dark . . . and I'll be back by ten or so . . . Ron will hardly miss me."

And that's pretty much how it went on Thursday. Love that girl. Nobody can make me forget my troubles better than Penny.

Thursday night, Penny calls at nine to prove it only took her three and a half hours to drive back to Chicago. This is good. Now I don't have to worry about her and I can go to bed. I'm setting the alarm for 4 A.M. I've been instructed to be at the hospital at six on Friday morning. There, I will meet Eve, who is being medic-bused from the nursing home to the hospital for the surgery. I'm more worried about me making it on time than I am about the operation. This is my first visit to Green Bay's brand new hospital. Dr. Brum has just relocated his office there.

Late as usual, I speed to Green Bay on Friday morning. At 6:05 A.M., I arrive at the hospital. It's so new there are no cars in the parking lot. I park in the first available spot next to handicapped. This must be my lucky day.

In the main reception area, I head for the desk to inquire if the medic-bus had arrived with Eve. Yes, it did. The driver took her up to pre-op ten minutes ago.

As I pause to catch my breath, I realize something odd is going on. I hear a piano playing Christmas carols. It's 6 A.M.! I turn around to look for the source. The main floor is immense. Not a soul is in sight . . . but I could swear . . . oh, there it is, way off in the corner, encircled by an audience of empty couches and cushy chairs. Yep, there it is, a grand piano—playing itself. The sight makes me shake the cobwebs out of my head. It's too early in the morning to appreciate the nuances of the 2001 version of a homey hospital.

I blindly follow the receptionist's directions to wherever Eve is. I know I'm there when I see another receptionist.

"Is my friend, Eve Kasper, here?" I ask her. Other than us, there's no one around.

"Oh, yes, I just wheeled her into the changing area. Tell me, is this her usual signature? She wasn't very talkative."

This woman isn't kidding. "Uh, yeah," I say. "Her signature is scrawled. That's because she can't write. She can't talk either. Eve had a brain aneurysm. Didn't the medic-bus driver sign her in, or give you instructions from the nursing home?"

The woman gulps. "Uh, maybe we'd better check on her. I left her alone . . . tossed her a gown and told her to change. She nodded yes. I thought she understood, so I closed the door . . ."

I'm gone. I run through the swinging door, frantically searching for Eve or staff or anyone. Finally, I find Eve, and the distraught receptionist has found us both. Eve is sitting in a wheelchair with her coat hanging off one arm and a half-unbuttoned blouse. She looks appropriately dazed.

"I'm so sorry," the receptionist gushes, and then retreats to from whence she came.

"Well, that's a fine how-do-you-do," I mutter. "I'm sorry, Eve. Got here as fast as I could. That woman didn't waste any time escaping. What makes her think I can do a better job than you have? I haven't a clue how to undress someone in a wheelchair. But, hey, I'm game to try. Wouldn't it be easier if we stood you up? Okay. Let's give this a try."

Standing in front of the wheelchair, I place my hands under her armpits—and lift. Ohhh. I think something snapped in my back, and Eve hasn't budged. "Okay, Eve, this time help me out. Ready? 1-2-3, lift." Eve bounces and weaves to no avail.

I can't cry uncle yet. Obviously, the receptionist thought I could do this. Maybe I don't have the knack because I haven't been a mother. I am so inept, I feel like half a woman.

"All right, Eve. One more time. Help me on 3. Ready? 1 . . . 2 . . . 3!" This time I grab her in a bear hug, lift, and stumble backward. Eureka. We're standing together. I'm exhausted.

"Okay. Let's start with the sweatpants." I hang on to Eve's back with one hand and find the waistband on the pants with the other hand, then try to pull the pants down. Obviously, nurses are born with three hands. How else could they do it? Eve is falling down; I have to hold her up and simultaneously pull down. I'm not double-jointed; I give up.

"Here, let's sit back down in the chair, Eve, and I'll go for help. Worthless, I'm just worthless. Sorry, Eve."

Eve's safely down and I open the door on what was a deserted room. However, now it's populated with two nurses and a doctor, excitedly chatting about the office Christmas party that afternoon.

"Excuse me," I interrupt. "I'm trying to help my friend in a wheelchair dress for her operation, and I can't do it alone. Could somebody help me, please?"

"Why, of course," the macho doctor responds. "You shouldn't be doing that anyway. Sue?" he says sternly.

Sue's first reaction is "who, me?" But she quickly recovers. "Of course, I'll do it, doctor. Kim, will you help?"

Oh, so that's the trick. Two nurses. I get it.

They're back in a flash. "She's on the bed resting," Sue says. "You can go back in now."

Soon after, Dr. Brum shows up. "Let's take another look at the scans," he says, waving me over. He brings them up rapidly on the computer monitor and begins clicking and rotating them. I don't know what I'm looking at and he apparently has forgotten I'm standing behind him. "Oh," he says. "Uh-oh. No good. Oh, I'd forgotten. Yes. So much blood. I don't know."

Uh-oh, not good? What the hell does that mean? "What's the matter?" I squeak.

"Oh, Donna," he says, finally realizing that I'm standing there. "I'm reviewing her brain scans. As you can see, there is a lot of blood on the brain, much more than I remembered. Look." He sweeps the picture on the monitor with his hand. I don't know what I'm looking at.

He turns on his stool and motions me to sit down. "Eve has a lot of blood and fluid on her brain. I don't know if this is going to work. But we have to give her a chance. Right?"

"Oh, sure," I respond. What happened to "piece of cake"? I think I'm going to be sick.

"Well, it's time to try. You wait in the waiting area. This will only take an hour. I'll come out afterward and let you know how the surgery went. Okay?"

I want to cry. I'm suddenly extremely exhausted. I can't do this, I think. Oh, quit whimpering, the little voice in my head says. Just do as you're told and buck up.

Back in the waiting room, a dozen or so brand-new sofas beckon. I choose the one farthest away from the ditzy receptionist, and almost instantly I'm "out" in some twilight zone of sleep. Then I'm visited by a bizarre and vivid dream.

In my dream, the waiting area is transformed into a funeral parlor and I'm seated on this couch. All of Eve's friends are lining up in front of me to offer their condolences. I chat and shake hands with each one. It feels so real. Suddenly, one of her friends is shaking my shoulder. Aggravated by the interruption, I turn to him, and snarl, "What?"

"Wake up, Donna," he says. "It's Dr. Brum. Come on, wake up. Eve's operation was a success."

"A success?" I ask groggily, not sure if I'm still dreaming.

He nods and smiles. "Go out for some breakfast. When you come back, you can see her. She'll still be out of it with the anesthesia, so don't expect to see any changes yet, maybe not even today. But you can visit with her for a little while. Now go get something to eat."

When I return to the hospital, Eve is alive and well, but very groggy. I desperately want to go home and sleep, so I kiss her goodbye and leave her with a promise to visit tomorrow.

# 11

# Merry Christmas!

Saturday morning I'm awakened by the pitter-patter-ping of sleet on the windows. Who'd believe it could be that warm on a Wisconsin winter day? (Ha-ha!) From my lakefront vantage point, it's difficult to tell what the ice storm is doing to the roadways. I flip on the radio to catch the news.

Apparently, America is still terrorized in the aftermath of 9/11. It's funny how I've barely given a thought to the state of the nation these two months. Prior to Eve's aneurysm, I was glued to one cable TV news channel or another. But just like a daytime soap opera, I can tune in months later to learn that nothing has changed.

Hmmm. I'll have to think about that later. The news is winding down; here comes the weather report.

"It's sunny outside, folks. High today in the twenties."

Well, that was informative. Guess I'll just call the hospital. If someone answers the phone, they should know what the driving conditions are like. Yep, it's sleeting in Green Bay. So I'm not budging from Baileys Harbor. "Could you please connect me to the neurosurgery nurses' station?" I ask. Nurse Lynn answers the phone.

"Hi," I say. "Are you, by any chance, Eve Kasper's nurse? Good. Well, this is her friend, Donna. How is she doing? Great. Say, could I ask a favor of you? Yesterday I told Eve I'd visit her today, but with the ice storm I can't make it. She won't have any other visitors. Now Eve probably won't comprehend what you say, but I'd appreciate it if you'd tell her that I'll see her tomorrow.

"What? Tell her myself? No, I don't think you understand. I'm talking about Eve Kasper. She doesn't know what a telephone is and, even if she did, Eve can't talk.

"What do you mean she's been talking your ear off all morning? Look, I think you have your patients mixed up. You only have two patients. Okey-dokey.

"Oh, no, no, please don't ring me through. No! Wait! Aargh! Damn!"

Now I'm pissed. I'm tapping my toe while I wait for Nurse Lynn to come back on the line and admit her big mistake. Stupid. Stupid. Finally the phone clicks and a voice comes across the line.

"Hi, Donna. Are you coming to visit me today?"

At that, my knees buckle and the blood drains from my head so quickly, I nearly faint. At first speechless, I finally manage to say, "Hi, it's Donna," which, of course, Eve already knows. "Well, hi. It's you, Eve." This is really sounding dumb. "I can hardly believe it's you.

"How are you feeling? Good. I'm sorry there's an ice storm. I would love to visit you. So you just keep talking to that nurse. Please tell her I'm sorry. Never mind why; she'll know. This is a miracle. Why? Oh, I'll tell you all about it someday, Eve. Maybe you should rest now. Yes, I'll see you tomorrow. I promise. Okay?"

As soon as I'm off the phone, I'm down on my knees to God, thanking Him/Her for my Christmas miracle. I'm truly stupefied. I never really expected to hear Eve's voice again. And that was Eve all right, not some brainless, robotic imitation. Glory be to the heavens!

On Sunday, I arrive at the hospital to find Eve sitting up in bed, wide-awake and waiting for me. I parade her around the hospital floor in a wheelchair and we talk about this and that for about an hour. Back in bed, she declares that she's tired. I stay on for another hour, watching her sleep, and finally decide to leave. But, before I do, I compare notes with the nurse. Today Eve was awake for four hours straight. It appears my New Year's wish has come true.

At last, it's Christmas Eve. I've made a reservation at a local motel that offers a free room to anyone visiting someone in a hospital over Christmas. Some day I intend to give that hotel chain's PR director a hug.

I arrive at the hospital late afternoon, having spent most of the day on the phone, updating half the world on Eve's progress. Disappointingly, Eve is difficult to rouse. At best, I can keep her awake for 15 minutes, and then she drifts off. I battle with myself as to whether I should call Dr. Brum. I decide to stuff my anxiety and not call, after talking with the nurse. She believes that the anesthesia, surgery, and effort to talk could all contribute to Eve's exhaustion.

I had brought a couple of wrapped presents, one for each of us, with the hope of making Christmas Eve festive. But it is not to be. I head downstairs to the hospital cafeteria. Tonight's holiday dinner is beef tips. The one server behind the counter offers to make up a tray that I can take back to Eve's room. How nice.

While I wait, I notice that the only other people in the cafeteria are two nurses on break, sitting by a Christmas tree. I understand that the hospital's brand new, but why does it have to be so empty? Oh, stuff the melodrama, Donna. I can't. A tear trickles down my cheek as I hand over a five-dollar bill for my meal to the server-turned-cashier. We wish each other a Merry Christmas. In my five-minute trek back to the room, I don't see another soul.

Back in Eve's room, which looks more like a four-star hotel suite than a hospital room, I enjoy a dinner so superb I would have willingly paid top dollar for it in a fancy restaurant. Eve's snoring now. I flip on the TV and catch an old Perry Como Christmas show in progress.

"Hey, Eve, wake up. It's one of our favorites. Perry's going to sing 'Ave Maria' pretty soon. Come on, please, Eve." Eve raises her eyelids to half-mast, smiles, and then down they go again. Oh well, oh hell. I stick around for another hour and then decide to call it a night.

Sure, it's only 7 P.M. But I'm wallowing in and out of self-pity. Since I can't seem to snap out of it, it's best just to go to bed. On the way to the hotel, I stop at a gas station and buy a package of cashews and a can of root beer. You never know, I might want a midnight snack.

I awake at 6 A.M. on Christmas morn with a tummy ache. Maybe the cashews weren't such a good idea. But then I open the drapes and sunlight pours into the room. It's a frosty, sparkling day and I'm filled with hope again. I dress in my new Christmas sweatshirt and jeans, and run down to the hotel office to express my sincere gratitude to the manager and to check out.

Hmmm, I should treat myself to breakfast. But what's open on Christmas? Well, duh, Denny's is always open. God bless Denny's.

After circling around Green Bay's hotel row a couple of times, I find it. There are cars in the parking lot. Whoopee. People. Inside, I note that they have an actual live Christmas tree in one corner. I can tell it's live because it's top-heavy and listing to one side. I ask to be seated next to it. A cheery young girl is my server. Next thing I know, I'm having a chitchat fit.

Without taking a breath, I compliment her on the tree, mention that I'm visiting my friend in the new hospital, and ask about her plans for Christmas. She's sweet enough to indulge me, returning often to fill my coffee cup. Finally, I'm finished. She asks if I'd like anything else.

I reply, "Yeah, it'd be nice to bring home a slice of pecan pie tonight. You know, comfort food."

She returns with the pie and my bill, and asks me to pay the cashier, then wishes me a Merry Christmas and disappears. I take the bill to figure the tip. There, at the bottom, I read "pecan pie, my treat, Merry Christmas."

Back at the hospital, I present Eve with a cardigan Christmas sweatshirt, ideal for warding off chills while I whiz her around the halls in a wheelchair. She presents me with a new coffee mug for the car. My old travel mug is worn out. We're thanking each other when who walks in but Santa himself, with one of his elves. Obviously, he wasn't told I would be there because I'm sure he would have brought me a present, too. After he leaves, I notice a couple of wrapped presents sitting on a table. They are from the nursing home. I really don't know how they got there . . . but Eve's making out like a bandit today. Am I jealous? Yes.

Mid-afternoon, Eve is pooping out. She's vastly improved over yesterday, so I'm okay with that. I tuck her in bed and head out with my coffee mug. I have some housecleaning waiting for me. Eve's friend, Liza, is coming to visit Wednesday through Friday, followed by Cass, Friday through Sunday. I sure hope they have presents for me.

Relatively speaking, the rest of the week "rocks." The doctor deems Eve ready for in-hospital rehabilitation, and she passes the hospital's rigid "swallowing" test. That means she can begin eating pureed foods. My appetite comes back and I actually enjoy dining out with friends again. Plus, I get presents.

Eve triumphantly returns to the nursing home on Friday and astounds the staff with her gift of gab. Spirits are high as New Year's Eve approaches. My one hope is to begin 2002 on a positive note by resolving the question of where to send Eve for her month of rehabilitation.

By the following Friday, I've narrowed my choices down to the Green Bay hospital where Eve had her coma, or a dedicated rehabilitation hospital in Chicago's western suburbs. With either hospital, my daytime presence is neither needed nor wanted. Visitors are encouraged to come around lunch, dinner, and evening hours. Of course, the caregiver receives some training, but that is scheduled for later in the month.

To my thinking, the one huge advantage Chicago holds over Green Bay is the visitor variety. Eve is a people person, and she shares many memories I know nothing about with her Chicago friends. I believe that that stimulation is necessary now.

To make Chicago a viable option, I'll need some help from Eve's hometown friends. First, I call Cass. She volunteers to coordinate the admission process and promises to share the caregiver role with me, and I can stay with her whenever I visit Eve. With Cass willing to help, I can manage the long-distance commute, a two-night stay, staff meetings, and visiting with Eve. I will be away only one full day so I won't worry about leaving the cats alone.

Penny calls in the middle of my planning session and offers to visit Eve daily at lunch. Mealtime coverage is important because Eve needs to be coaxed into eating 2,000 calories' worth of unappetizing mush a day. Otherwise, the powers-that-be won't remove the feeding tube.

Before I know it, Eve has a bed reserved for January 8 in the Chicago-area rehab. By January 7, I'm packing Eve's clothes at the nursing home. The next day, we say our good-byes to the nurses and aides. As I'm gushing with gratitude to the nursing home owner, she says, "You have no idea what Eve's presence has done for the morale of the staff. We want to thank both of you." We hug.

And off Eve and I go to Chicago.

# 12

# Happy New Year?

With careful planning, the five-hour trip to Chicago goes without a hitch, even with three stops along the way to ensure Eve's continence. Thank you, State of Wisconsin, for maintaining such pristine public rest rooms.

When we arrive at the entrance to the rehabilitation hospital, Cass is there to greet us. When she opens Eve's car door, both Cass and I learn that Eve's first road trip has made her carsick. I think Cass was expecting a hug instead.

Cass races into the hospital to find someone to help Eve in and, I hope, take her to a room, while I monkey around with the admissions process. At the end of the intake interview, the caseworker, Lois, asks me what my rehabilitation goals are for Eve.

I resist the urge to quip, "Well, I want you to fix her, duh." Instead, I say, "Please teach her to eat, remove that feeding tube, and help her regain continence." In my naïveté, I expect that these goals are pretty obvious and will be accomplished with the institutional "left hand" while the "right hand" is doing the tricky stuff like teaching Eve how to bathe, talk, walk, and plan a daily routine.

After the hour interview, I set out to find Cass who, I presume, is with Eve in her room. When I reach the room, I notice a warning sign posted on the door: "Caution. Occupant has a highly contagious disease."

Oh, my God. I burst into the room, wondering what exotic disease Eve picked up during the car ride. Eve's in bed, sleeping, and Cass is reading a magazine. I note that the curtain is drawn, splitting off Eve's half of the room.

"What's with Eve?" I whisper, as I'm pointing at the sign. "I thought she was just carsick."

"Nothing's wrong with Eve," Cass responds. "But I don't believe her roommate's in the pink, as they say."

Quickly, my temper emerges and races to catch up with my pulse. "Eve's roommate has a contagious disease? Are these people blanking nuts? Don't I have enough of a mess?" My whisper is turning into a series of squeaks, and Cass is trying unsuccessfully to clamp a hand over my mouth.

"Look, Donna, I'm sure the nurses' station will be able to explain. Why don't you ask?" Then she pauses. "On second thought, let me do the asking. I'm going with you. Please stay calm, for me?"

While standing at the nurses' station, listening to Cass blah-blah-blah with the nurse, I have one of those premonitions that starts as a tummy rumble. This hospital is not very customer-oriented. It appears no amount of polite complaining is going to change the minds of a staff that has only one hour left until shift change.

On the way back to Eve's room, I fake a calm attitude. "So," I say, "let me restate what I heard the nurse tell you. Eve's roommate has uncontrollable diarrhea, which has something highly contagious in it, but they don't know what it is. However, as soon as her son or daughter gets here, which may be tomorrow, the woman will be taken to a regular hospital to—well, you tell me, Cass—to die or something? Meanwhile, she's Eve's roommate. There are no other beds available. Did you get a good look at that staff? Can't you just picture them all drawing straws to see who enters this room at their own risk?" Finally, I sputter to a halt.

Cass shrugs and gives me one of those "you're dramatizing, Donna, stop it" looks. Her nonchalance sends me careening toward rage.

Thankfully, a sudden insight stops me from lashing out. This rehab hospital stay is Cass's baby, not mine. She'll be handling more of the day-to-day than I will. She's Eve's friend, too. Oh, man, I'm going to have to be diplomatic here, a trait no one ever accuses me of possessing.

"Okay, Cass. I'll take it easy. It's way beyond my control anyway. Let's go out for an early dinner somewhere in the neighborhood. Then we can sit with Eve till the end of visiting hours. Hope she wakes up for a little while."

And thus begins Eve's much-prayed-for rehabilitation program. As "they" say, be careful what you pray for. On my three-day-a-week visits, I find myself in big-city-hospital culture shock more often than not. It's so impersonal. So into assembly-line technique. So very uninspiring. On my long treks back to Door County, I spend my day-dream time wondering how in the world these rehab techniques will work in the home situation. But then, maybe they want me to think this brain rehab is the sole domain of the professionals. It sure seems that way.

Overshadowing my negative gut-level reaction to the environment is the incredible parade of friends who regularly visit Eve. On the days I'm not there, Penny and Cass are, without fail. Cass even takes home Eve's laundry. Penny and Cass bring Eve to their homes on alternating Sundays for a family-style dinner.

Liza also visits several times, bringing fancy ice cream, dominoes, and Yahtzee. I often hear how three or four of Eve's assorted friends have stayed the entire evening to talk and play games with her. Even our former Naperville hairdresser visits one night, toting a portable haircut kit. With his usual magic touch, he transforms Eve's postoperation hair disaster into a beautiful "do." Sometimes, relatives of Eve's friends visit. For instance, Penny's sister stops by several times after work. And Cass's nephew brings his dog on "pet" day. Judging from the light returning to Eve's eyes, the Chicago rehabilitation period is an astounding success, thanks to her friends.

Clinically speaking, the experience is disappointing—verging on disastrous, for me. I'm having nightmares as I count the days until I will be the sole caregiver. Oh, sure, the hospital therapists teach us how to manage the shower-for-two, how to monitor her calorie count, climbing stairs, getting in a car, and some other practicalities. But I am terribly distressed by their refusal to remove the feeding tube. They say it's because they can't be sure I can manage to persuade Eve to eat 2,000 calories a day at home. I say they're protecting themselves from whatever.

Eve's limited continence training, which was begun at the nursing home, completely unravels at the hospital. No matter how much I beg, scream, and plead, all the way up the "nursing chain" to the director, the staff never institutes a daily potty-training routine. More than once, I arrive from Wisconsin to find Eve sitting in a mess in the middle of a therapy session. I guess the therapists don't consider it their job to take Eve to the bathroom during sessions and, of course, the nurses are never around to help.

By the time Eve is discharged, my emotional reactions are a mix of disgruntled dismay with the hospital and eternal gratitude to Eve's friends.

On the last day, Eve's caseworker, who now makes it a habit to avoid me, stops in Eve's room to talk. She begins, "This is highly unusual, but Eve's insurance caseworker called me yesterday. You're to contact NEW. That's the Northeast Wisconsin Curative Rehabilitation Center. The insurance company has worked out a plan with NEW for Eve's continued rehab, which you may find very interesting. Call this number tomorrow to set up an appointment with their admissions director." She hands me a card.

After our chat, I resume packing up Eve's room. Next thing I know, an orderly comes waltzing in with a wheelchair.

Ignoring my presence, he says to Eve, "Here's the wheelchair you ordered for home care. We've put the charge on your hospital bill."

Eve smiles and nods.

"Whoa, not so fast," I halt him. "Wait just a second." Words, smoke, and, perhaps, fire are spewing from my mouth. "You're saying this wheelchair was ordered by her? A person with brain damage? Why was it never discussed with me? We live in a home, not a hospital with 10-foot-wide hallways. Who 'sold' her this bill of goods?"

He shakes his head. "Uh, I don't know, lady. I'm just delivering it."

"Well, undeliver it, and hand me that clipboard so I can write 'Refused' in real big letters."

Just then the caseworker makes another appearance. We review the situation together.

"Look," I say, "when Eve left the nursing home she was walking with my assistance. No walker, no wheelchair. The nurses' aides explained to me that the therapist didn't want Eve dependent on walking aids. Now you're telling me she needs a wheelchair to negotiate the house after a month in a fancy rehabilitation hospital?

"Anyway, according to this bill, it's going to cost me big bucks to boot. No way. Back where I come from—rural Wisconsin—we have a program that will lend us a free wheelchair, but only if we need one, which we don't. Thank you, but we're going home without a wheelchair or a walker, or any other crutches. Sheesh."

The caseworker simply nods agreeably, no doubt counting the moments until Eve is discharged and I go away.

"So, that's rehab Chicago-style," I mumble to Eve as I roll her out to the car. "All I can say is, I'm glad your friends visited." Eve smiles and nods . . . and then we're on our way back.

# PART TWO

# RIDING THE ROLLER COASTER TO RECOVERY

# Introduction

At this point in our lives, I never dreamed I'd be writing a book about Eve's successful recovery. Quite frankly, I was simply caregiving by the "seat of my pants."

Consequently, all of the rehabilitation techniques I tried with Eve were not scientifically documented; the variables were not controlled and the results were not faithfully recorded. I am one caregiver; Eve is one survivor. There are dozens of uncontrolled variables that affect our daily lives. Taken altogether, we do not "prove" anything. Our experience may give you food for thought, however.

For the most part, I developed my rehabilitation program using concepts from three semi-scientific disciplines: advertising, the 12-Step program, and subconscious persuasion methods for changing behaviors. I say semi-scientific because all three are operating "theories" of behavior motivation and modification. In other words, no scientists have proven their success beyond doubt, but the anecdotal evidence suggests they are successful in certain areas.

I have intertwined all three theories in my method. In the following pages, I tell and show to the best of my ability everything I did. I am not sure exactly what worked, when, or why. I was operating primarily on intuition, meaning if I thought something was working, I tried it again.

Probably, the one variable I did control was that I didn't give up easily on any technique. From the very start, I gave myself a two-year time limit to keep trying whatever came to my mind as rehabilitation, regardless of Eve's response or anyone's judgment of success (including my own). I always opted in favor of "Try it again."

It will simplify things if you keep in mind that advertising and the 12-Step program are both variations of subconscious communication and suggestion methods. Advertising appeals to subconscious needs and desires using the simple, emotional language that captures the subconscious mind's attention. The 12-Step program uses positive action to "teach" the subconscious mind that a new behavior is desirable and beneficial for a person's survival.

Both disciplines attempt to bypass the analytical conscious mind. Both try to alleviate the stresses of life by compartmentalizing life into manageable segments. The 12-Step program does it with constant reminders to live "one day at a time." Advertising encapsulates its messages in one-minute daydream scenarios called commercials, or on a magazine page filled with pictures and words. Both are designed to create the ideal environment for the motivating sales message.

You do not have to be a master of any of these disciplines to understand or experiment with any of the approaches I used with Eve. You've done some of these things automatically; others fall into the category of old-fashioned common sense. What I hope to accomplish here is to tell you why some of the things you've done are working and to inspire you to keep doing them, whether or not you see immediate results.

As your cheerleader, I am also encouraging you to go "over the top" with emotional appeals for behavioral change aimed at reaching the survivor's subconscious mind. At the same time, I am cautioning you not to harbor unrealistic expectations of immediate success.

For your own mental health and emotional stability, remember that the brain will heal at its own rate. We, the caregivers, are just providing the "right" direction and a fertile environment for experiential learning.

By and by, you'll see how we caregivers also require retraining ourselves. We need to find our own power in a mostly chaotic environment where our lives are spent waiting for a response from the survivor. We need to cultivate a relaxed, receptive demeanor, using whatever tools of relaxation are out there. We also need to motivate ourselves to adapt to the mostly boring, frustrating, and mundane routine of daily brain rehabilitation.

We need to teach, yet not enmesh ourselves with the survivor or become dependent on a certain outcome to light up our lives. Incidentally, for no-nonsense advice in this area, make the acquaintance of an Al-Anon member. Al-Anons are the experts in detaching with love. They know all the pitfalls of codependency, enabling, and the emotionally painful consequences of harboring unrealistic expectations.

When you read my stories, my examples, you may be tempted to dismiss them because they don't match your specific situation. Believe me, I realize every stroke, every brain incident, is different. I've seen that disqualifier on many a rehab or support website and in home therapy books. Yes, they are all different. But I'm inviting you to look for the similarities between your case and mine.

This is what the entire 12-Step program teaching method is based on. One member shares a story. We, the listeners, look for the similarities, take the lessons we need to hear, and leave the rest on the table. That's how recovery happens in a roomful of "misfit" recovering souls with diverse backgrounds: ministers, streetwalkers, lawyers, laborers, doctors, artists, house painters, high school kids, and octogenarian retirees. If you read about my experience with an open mind, you'll be amazed not only at the similarities, but also at the rehabilitation strategies you will be inspired to create and try in your own particular circumstances.

# 13

# In Search of Serenity

I've never heard of NEW (Northeast Wisconsin) Brain Rehabilitation Center, but then, why would I? Before I make the appointment, I call Marie at the nursing home to get the lowdown on it. She's helped me several times over the past month to cope with Eve's disappointing rehabilitation routine. During the conversation, she mentions that she conveyed my disenchantment with the Chicago rehab in a follow-up call with her telephone "buddy," Eve's insurance caseworker. NEW was their brainchild in a continuing effort to help me as best they could.

Per Eve's insurance policy, she is entitled to three hours of outpatient rehabilitation for ten weeks. I really had no clue where to take Eve for rehab, except I knew there was some sort of therapy clinic in close-by Sturgeon Bay.

During my appointment at NEW, Harriet, the admissions director, says, "The insurance company has struck a deal with us to provide the total outpatient program for Eve."

"Oh," I mumble, "I can hardly wait to hear this one."

Harriet smiles at me. It's a special smile, just for beleaguered caregivers. "No, you're going to like this, Donna. We can provide Eve with three one-hour occupational, physical, and speech therapy sessions three days a week for ten weeks."

I blanch. "You mean I have to drive all this way for a one-hour session three days a week?"

"No, you're not listening. Three one-hour sessions each day, three days a week, for ten weeks. It's all worked out. Plus I might throw in a priority management skills class, if you'll agree to stay at Eve's side between sessions. I don't think she's capable of finding her way around without assistance. We can do this if you'll assume responsibility for her."

"Oh, you betcha," I say. "Did God send you down from heaven? Geez, thank you. And that wonderful nursing home . . . and the insurance company?" (I can hardly believe I'm actually grateful to the insurance company.) "Wow. It's a deal. When do we start?"

She says, "Monday we have evaluations; we'll schedule Eve for therapy Wednesday and Friday next week. See you and Eve at 8:30?"

"With bells on Eve's toes," I reply.

On the way back from our NEW admissions meeting, our car whizzes by the "Welcome to Door County" sign that always elicited an "Ah, we're home" spoken in unison. Instead of relief, I feel a tear trickle down my cheek.

I should be happy. Eve is finally sitting next to me. I should be grateful we've still got a home to go to. I should be hopeful that NEW can work wonders with Eve's disabilities. I am not.

Instead, my mind has raced through the worry stage and is now well on its way to fear of the unknown. I don't know what to do, so I guess I'll pray.

"God, grant me the serenity to accept the things I cannot change, courage to change the things I can, and the wisdom to know the difference."

I continue driving. I am waiting for an answer. Nothing. I feel like my prayer has been ignored and that the deities have abandoned me.

"Oh, screw it," I say. Then, ignoring my own pitiful pain, I turn to Eve and ask her how she's feeling. That works. Yep, now that I stopped feeling sorry for myself, serenity is slowly dribbling into my soul.

As I continue driving, a thought pops into my head. What if I already have all the tools I need for rehabilitating Eve? As for the plan, maybe that will come to me over time. I'm too tired to execute a plan today . . . and anyway, I'm not sure I even understand the problem.

I chuckle. Of course, no matter what the problem is, I can bet it involves me. And I do know that if the "old" Eve could somehow magically appear on the front seat next to me, all my troubles would disappear. Duh. Then that must be the problem, dopey: how to bring back the "old" Eve.

And sure as shooting, that involves me. I live with her, for Pete's sake.

Okay, then according to my 12-Step training, if I am part of the problem, then I am also part of the solution. And as usual, the solution requires change. Since I am powerless to change Eve (and so is she), then all I can do is change myself.

Well, that wisdom works in most problem situations, but truly I don't see how my changing will help "fix" Eve. Perhaps I lack perception here because I haven't changed enough to know what's wrong with me in this whole brain trauma caregiving situation.

Oh, rats. Let me guess, God. Darn, I probably haven't fully accepted how very powerless I am to fix Eve. That's why my mind is so messed up.

Apparently, I've bought into our society's never-ending quest for the quick fix. Yep, I'll bet I believe that a few little physical/occupational/ speech therapy sessions will make it all better. But whether those sessions work or not, they won't solve the problem as I see it: How do I bring back the heart, soul, and personality of my friend? Those therapies don't even address that issue. So how can they solve the problem?

In actuality, I am probably the only person able and willing to try to bring Eve back. But I have no clue how to do it. If my problem is lack of knowledge and training, then I have to focus on fixing me to assume my new role.

Would it help me to go to school? No, there are no courses in heart and soul brain rehabilitation. Anyway, I know enough about Eve to fill a book. Then that's not my problem, nor the solution.

Perhaps I'll just have to sit and wait for Eve to reveal the "problem" and all of its aspects in the home caregiving situation. As I interrelate with her on a daily basis, living in the scenario, then more of the problem, and hence the solution, will be revealed.

Meanwhile, I better work on practicing patience and accepting that most of what I will be doing immediately is mastering the physical aspects of caregiving. I'll simply have to accept that I need to establish a caregiving routine and get enough experience in things like feeding and bathing Eve so that my confidence in performing these tasks is no longer an issue. Then perhaps I can focus on what I believe is the real problem here: how to bring back the essence of Eve.

Just working on my role as part of the problem seems mind-boggling to me. I better do what the program suggests: I will take things one day at a time (maybe an hour at a time) until I am more comfortable with my role in the situation.

After I've gotten Eve to a point where she can bathe and feed herself, I can do some thinking about this heart and soul idea. All of a sudden a selfish little thought pops into my head: Maybe I can skip over the nasty parts and jump right into the heart and soul of my rehabilitation plan. I'm chuckling now. There you go, Donna, always looking for the easy way out. Lord, give me patience, right away.

Mind games . . . how I love to play them. And this might be the highest stakes mind game of my life.

As a creative advertising writer, I have been paid to play mind games my entire career. Now that I'm away from the scene, I am an avid armchair critic of those one-minute sales messages that appear nightly on the tube.

Usually the best commercials are the slickest. They are the ones that entertain as they stimulate our deepest desires and needs, then cleverly associate the satisfaction of that need or desire with the product. The formula goes something like this: beautiful girl/macho car/sexual innuendo, or hungry family/cake mix/appreciation of Mom. It is the science of indirect subconscious suggestion elevated to an art.

Crafty advertisers will use anything to attract attention and hold it. Pretty scenery, sexy models, smiling babies, outlandish humor, ridiculous puns, loud irritating noises, and repetition. All are aimed at bypassing the conscious mind and waking up those subconscious needs. Appropriately, most commercials are written simply and at a level a child can understand—just the way our subconscious minds "think."

So why not use these same techniques to deliver my messages to Eve? Instructions on personal hygiene, safety in the home, eating and cleaning up after herself. In her case, I won't have to worry about getting through the ever-analyzing conscious mind, so my messages might have some real impact. This whole process, of course, requires that I communicate with her. Right now, she doesn't converse and doesn't always comprehend what I say. I can't hold her attention for a long enough period of time to get my "advertising" messages across. Hmmm, I'll have to think some more about that.

"Hey, Eve, wake up. We're home."

Whew. We've both survived our first week of therapy at NEW. Now it's Saturday and I'm finally enjoying coffee again, with too many cigarettes. From my vantage point at the dining room table, I'm looking out across a snow-blanketed backyard at frozen Baileys Harbor, Lake Michigan, and beyond. Naked birches with black bark slashings offer a most interesting contrast to the pearly white-on-white world. I feel like the view—frozen in time and space.

Whatever became of the blue? I wonder.

It's a faded memory, like Eve, who is sitting next to me, slurping her oatmeal. She gulps her orange juice; I remind her to slow down. My mood is as bleak as the day. What am I going to do?

Talk about a clueless caregiver; it's taken all of my energy this week just to barely manage the house, bills, and Eve's rehabilitation routine. I damn my own inadequacies. I'm a daydreamer, a creative muser, an idea person. When it comes to household tasks, I'm not very efficient or motivated. In fact, I'm downright lazy. Donna abhors the one thing Eve needs the most: routine. I'm frightened by my future. The simplest caregiving chores are already frustrating me, calling me into a life I never, ever wanted. Boring, mundane routine.

Oh well, I chastise myself, you've been on a seven-year vacation from the monotony of everyday living. Surprise. It's time to pay the piper. Better get off your duff and begin this day, or you'll soon be looking at dinnertime without a supply of groceries. But first, "Let's go shower, Eve. Gotta take care of some bad business."

Yesterday, at NEW, the resident nurse stopped in at one of the therapy sessions to do a quick health check on Eve. "What about this feeding tube?" she asked.

"Oh, I'm on top of that," I replied. "The doctor who put it in is going to take it out next week."

She gave me one of those "you are just too stupid" looks. "Fine," she retorted, "but meanwhile you might try cleaning it."

"Do what?" Yuck. Man, am I stupid. Another instance of ignoring what I don't want to do! I'm hoping against hope that she'll feel sorry for me and do it herself. Then the old manipulative me takes over. "But I don't know how," I say, with my best "helpless" look.

"Well, you'd better learn soon. Like, do it when you give her the next shower, in case you make a mess." I note that she's avoiding my imploring gaze. "Look," she says, throwing me a bone, "I'll explain how to do it. Take notes, if you wish."

Honestly, I really tried to listen and take notes, but my mind kept going blank. I noted that the explanation was riddled with cautions, however. Better do this when I'm awake.

The moment of truth has arrived. I position Eve in front of the bathroom sink and strip her. My first mistake is not stripping me.

Damn, I realize I forgot to bring the instructions with me. My second mistake is fooling myself that I can remember how to do this without them. Wrong. I no sooner start the cleaning process when—surprise—the tube assumes a life of its own, spraying its contents all over Eve, my nightgown and robe, the cabinets and the floor. Lord, what a disgusting mess.

"Guess I should have pinched that tube," I say.

Eve smiles and nods. "Yes, you should have."

"Oh, thanks, Eve. Now you find your tongue," I sputter angrily, and then quickly apologize. This is your stupidity in action, I admonish myself. Don't take it out on the patient. Well, I can clean up the rest of this mess later. Right now, Eve's wearing yesterday's dinner and so am I.

I turn on the faucet and we step into the shower. As the water sprays us, Eve fights me. Like many stroke victims, Eve hates that feeling of shower water beating on her head. As I'm rinsing the shampoo residue, she spastically dodges the drips, while I'm trying to maintain our footing and balance in the too-small shower stall. Luckily, our shower has a built-in bench and a handheld spray. I force her to sit. If I let her hold my hand while I spray her, she appears to calm down a little. The trade-off is that she gets cold more quickly at this far end of the shower. She's shivering violently now.

I work as fast as I can to clean and rinse her. Finally, she's finished and we step out of the shower. I wrap Eve in a giant towel and seat her on the toilet under the heat fan and next to the portable heater. Her teeth stop chattering, but I'm freezing my fanny off . . . and still unclean.

"Don't move," I command, as I bounce back into the shower. Shampoo pours into my eyes, which are wide open in order to keep an eye on Eve. "Damn," I curse myself, wondering which body parts I can skip so that I can get out of this shower and attend to Eve. I fear she'll catch a cold, or worse yet, the flu, if she gets a chill.

Presto. I'm as clean as I am going to be. The iron-hard water hasn't cleanly rinsed my hair, but who cares? Ignoring my own goose bumps, I jump out of the shower and vigorously towel-dry Eve tip-top to toes. Then I whip out the blow-dryer and try to make styling sense out of Eve's erratic hairdo. She's sensitive to the heat, too, so she's shaking her head while I'm fighting to hold it still.

Ta-dah! The ordeal is finally over. I survey the results. Eve's cowlick is standing straight up; she looks like a drugged rooster. My own partially dry hair doesn't look much better. I'm exhausted and fighting back tears as I pick up my soiled robe and head for the laundry. It's only 9 A.M. While the washing machine churns, I fill a pail with Pine Sol to clean up the feed tube debris on the bathroom floor. Really clueless.

Half an hour later, I have finished mopping the floor and over-dressing Eve. She is sitting at the dining room table again, wrapped in an afghan to protect her against any wayward drafts. I'm working on a grocery shopping list. Hamburgers, hot dogs, tuna fish, and ham and eggs. I could live with that. I'll just toss in a salad and fruit for dessert and, voila, the four food group requirements are satisfied. Oh yeah, don't want to forget to buy more ice cream for the dairy group. If I strategically rotate the meals, Eve will never notice. There is a benefit to her short-term memory loss, after all.

My mind jokes aren't working too well, as I watch a wayward teardrop stain my shopping list. Stop it, I caution myself. You can't afford even a momentary exercise in self-pity. You know the old A.A. adage: "Poor me! Poor Me! Pour me a drink!" It's dangerous territory, so "Quit it," I mutter aloud.

"What did you say?" asks Eve. She's looking at me with those glazed, dopey eyes. My tears momentarily blind me.

"Nothing. Never mind, Eve." I can feel myself going down when, whoopee, the phone rings.

It's my A.A. sponsor, Yolanda, calling to find out why I haven't called her. "Because I'm wallowing in self-pity," I respond with sarcasm aimed at myself. I brace myself for the tongue-lashing I've obviously asked for.

It's difficult to describe the "mature" sponsor-sponsee relationship. It's not like friendship, or a mother-daughter (or father-son) relationship, and not a psychologist-patient relationship. It's a relationship based on the mutual goal of recovery. There is a payoff for both parties in the process.

In the process of working the program steps, the sponsee has revealed her deepest, darkest secrets to the sponsor, as well as habitual behavior patterns and defense mechanisms the sponsee uses, mostly unsuccessfully, to deal with her life. Armed with this knowledge, the sponsor can offer the sponsee a suggestion on how she might solve her current problem or deal with her emotional pain by changing her behavior or attitude, or both. The basis for the sponsor's suggestion is usually a program step or concept that the sponsor has learned from her own experience. In the end, the sponsee has a new direction to follow, if she chooses. The payoff for the sponsor is that her program receives a booster shot, because she has reinforced the principles that her own program is based on—whether or not the sponsee follows the direction.

It's not therapy, not advice, and initially not usually very comforting for the pained sponsee. But it's a 24/7 support system that works in good times and bad, including life-and-death situations.

And now I await the reprimand I assume I deserve after making the flippant remark about my state of serenity deteriorating into self-pity. As usual, I "guess" wrong about my sponsor's reaction. Instead of a sermon, I hear a calm, soothing voice delivering words of comfort—and hope?

"Come on, kid, you've been through some really tough times before. Need I remind you of when you were broke, losing your condo, no job in sight? And, worst of all, the booze had taken away your mind. That beautiful creative mind you prized so highly. Do you remember what I told you then?"

"Oh, you bet I do. You told me to wash the windows, mop the floor, and then go to an A.A. meeting. Big help you were!" I laugh for the first time all day.

"And so, what's on the agenda today . . . cleaning ovens or toilets?" Yolanda asks, in an obvious maneuver to keep me off my pity-pot.

"Well, I already cleaned up the total disaster of our personal hygiene exercise. Now I'm finishing up the shopping list for a week's worth of mouth-watering gourmet meals. Geez, why didn't you ever teach me how to cook?"

"Because I wasn't your mother 13 years ago and I'm not gonna be now. And don't ever think you can manipulate me. You're an amateur compared to me."

Nice shot. Score one for the sponsor.

"Anyway, Donna, why don't we take a moment here to review the 12-Step program? Try this one on for size. Donna is powerless over the caregiving situation with Eve, and her life is totally unmanageable."

"You're telling me," I sarcastically reply.

"Shut up," she says. "Let's cut the angry sarcasm and get right to the part where you start listening to me. Are you teachable yet?"

"Yes, ma'm," I humbly reply. That woman has such a way with words.

"Okay. You've admitted you're powerless. Why don't you try accepting that fact right now? After all, there is a big difference between acceptance and sorrowful resignation, isn't there?" She continues, "I believe I'm quoting you now."

"Uh-huh." Got me again, I see.

"Okay. So you've accepted you're powerless. Remember the slogan: I can't, He can, so let Him! Why don't you tell me where you are at with your Higher Power? Did you ask Him/Her/Whomever for help today? Don't answer me; 'cause you obviously haven't had a chance to meditate this morning, right?"

I have no intention of answering her.

She continues, "Your only task today, my dear, is to keep doing the next right thing. Everything else should be turned over to the care of your Higher Power. That includes how well you perform your caregiver tasks. You just do your best and leave the outcome to your Higher Power. And no expectations, for Eve or for yourself. How in the world can you expect to handle this as efficiently as a nurse when you've never done these things before? 'Remember, your life is none of your business.'"

Oh, there's that nonsensical slogan she's always tossing out at me. "I don't get it," I say.

"Get this," she retaliates. "If you allow yourself to go crazy, who's going to take care of you?"

"You?" I respond hopefully.

"No, I'm not taking care of a pain in the butt like you. I've coddled you for too many years already."

Coddled me? I don't think so.

"Now, tell me, can I please speak to the sober Donna who used to work a program?"

"Yeah, yeah, yeah."

"Write this down. The same God who cares for you also cares for Eve. He's not going to let you kill her after all you've been through to keep her alive. Trust me on this. Now I want you to lighten up. When you're out at the store, stop somewhere and rent a movie for tonight. By the way, what are you going to do with Eve while you're at the store? Tie her up in bed?"

"Oh, damn, I haven't really thought that through. I guess I'll leave her in the car."

"With the engine running for heat?"

Immediately, I'm visited by a vision of confused, dopey Eve sliding behind the wheel and taking off for God knows where to escape the tyranny of my caregiving. "Not such a good idea, I guess. Maybe I'll see if there's anything in the freezer." I offer a silent prayer for a TV dinner or two as I carry the phone into the kitchen. "Oh, thank God," I bless the phone. "It's like the miracle of the loaves and the fishes. I have two frozen lasagnas and two chicken pot pies. Where'd they come from? They've got to be six months old."

"Now, Donna, what have we learned from this mini-crisis?" Yolanda asks.

"That I better stock up on ice cream 'cause we don't have enough of that for the weekend," I reply. Luckily, my sponsor chuckles.

"How about doing your grocery shopping while Eve's occupied with her rehabilitation therapy? They do have grocery stores in Green Bay, I presume? Now let this be a lesson to you. If you'd stop spinning long enough to work a program, and perhaps pray the Serenity Prayer on occasion, you'll start thinking and stop reacting to situations. Serenity is not an option here. You need it to survive, Donna."

"I get the message. Thank you once again."

"Next time, don't forget to call your sponsor when your panic begins. Better yet, keep your expectation level low and there'll be nothing to panic about."

Right, no expectations. I knew that, didn't I? "Thanks for the reminder. Don't get too comfortable. You'll probably be hearing from me soon. Bye-bye, for now."

I hang up the phone with a grumble . . . and the intuitive thought that too-quiet Eve must have fallen asleep at the dining room table. Time for a late morning nap. With Eve safely tucked away, I toss in another load of laundry and turn my attention to the teetering tower of unopened medical bills and insurance statements, most of which I have successfully ignored for several weeks now. As I rip open the envelopes and peruse their contents, my tummy lurches toward nausea. The words "Exceeds usual and customary charges"— the synonym for financial disaster—greet me on nearly every page.

Oh, man, I thought insurance was covering this after the deductible. But they're weaseling out of everything they can. Oh boy, we're in big trouble now. "And so," I say aloud, so that I'll hear it, "what did you expect?"

Worse yet, it appears that all the big providers are covered, while the little labs and one-time doctors seem to have fallen into the deductible area. That leaves me with no leverage to bargain for low monthly payment plans. These little guys want to be paid every-thing—like last month. How am I going to do this? Oh, barf.

I feel clouds of panic swirling in my brain again. I dare not call my sponsor; she'll disown me. It hasn't even been an hour since her phone call. I've got to quiet down. Maybe I'll pray . . . on my knees this time.

In time, the calm comes. Sure, my life is unmanageable on almost every front. But I've been there before . . . and with less sobri-ety under my belt than I have now. What I did then, I can do again. Turn the whole sorry mess over to my Higher Power's care. Then proceed to do the next right thing. Even if I don't know what I'm doing, I can "act as if" I do. Action is good. Anxiety has a hard time dragging down a moving target. And, how about that trusty serenity tool I used to practice all the time—cultivating an attitude of gratitude?

Today, we have food, shelter, clothing . . . even if it is frozen, overfinanced, and unfashionable. Best of all, Eve is not a vegetable. I don't have to flip her over every three hours to guard against bedsores. We've made some progress. Who says there isn't room for more?

But what will I do with Eve? None of this helps me with Eve. I can't even communicate with her. I feel my serenity slipping away. No. Wait. Let's see. If I can't communicate with her normally, maybe I can try abnormally. Chuckle. I made a joke. That's it, lighten up a little. Now let's see, what abnormal communication mode can I use? Thought transference? ESP? Drums? Oh hell, I surrender. Yep. I'm going to give up now. You hear that, God? I'm ready to let go . . . any minute now.

Oh, for crying out loud. You're going bats. Just relax. Come on. Count backward from ten to one and ask your subconscious to come to the rescue.

Wait a second. Subconscious. Did any doctor say Eve's subconscious was damaged? Oh, don't be dumb. You know most of them think subconscious communication is one step beyond voodoo magic.

But I don't think so, do I? I know it's worked for me. For sure, I've used it in advertising. If I can just get Eve to pay attention to me, then maybe—just maybe—I can use those advertising techniques to ask her subconscious to help heal her brain.

That's crazy. So what? I'm going crazy anyway. We're both going down with a sinking ship. I need a pencil and paper. I'm going to write a letter to myself and explain how this could work. What the hell else am I doing anyway? It's worth a shot.

# 14

# Exploring the Subconscious

I first met up with the subconscious mind in one of my college advertising classes. The professor explained to the fledgling copywriters that the most powerful ads employ emotional appeals that are aligned with a person's subconscious value system. It was our job as copywriters to identify a need, match it with a subconscious value, then show how the advertised product would satisfy that need and reinforce the value.

Our advertising lesson was based on a popular psychology theory known as Maslow's hierarchy of values. As the professor pointed out, above and beyond the basic needs for food, shelter, and clothing, a whole slew of values cry out for satisfaction. These values, the source of self-esteem, include the well-being of the family, meaningful work, artistic expression, good health, thirst for knowledge, physical attractiveness, and so on.

Thus we learned to create ads based on the hierarchy of values.

For example, an ad for a packaged cake mix went beyond the food value of the cake to appeal to the homemaker's desire to please her husband and delight her children by serving a homemade dessert. An ad for luxury cars ignored engineering-speak and instead appealed to a man's desire to show off his success as the family breadwinner. Over the years, the sales results for popular products have proven the phenomenal success of advertisements based on appeals to the value system that exists in the subconscious minds of American consumers.

Fast-forward to my late twenties, when I signed up for one of those adult evening education classes that promised I could "Learn to Relax Using Creative Visualization Techniques." Here I learned another valuable lesson about the subconscious: its power to change my feelings, my thoughts, and therefore my actions. Though I was still relatively young, I was not immune to career burnout, a risk one takes in the high-pressure ad biz. Much to my dismay, I was experiencing high anxiety every time I stood up to speak in a sales meeting. It baffled me—and defied my self-talk to "Go away!" I never used to be afraid of an audience. But that knowledge, even combined with occasional successful experiences, couldn't override the ever-increasing, gut-wrenching fear that gripped me in business meetings. I needed relief—fast, fast, fast.

Amazingly enough, the simple creative visualization exercises I learned in those night classes eventually helped me calm down on the job. At first, I thought the teacher was a magician. But when we became friends, I discovered just how practical and reality-based she was. A former teacher turned homemaker, my friend explained that she originally learned these techniques to combat headaches born of her own anxious personality. Nothing mysterious about it. She was simply spreading the good news. Over the next few years, she taught me various ways to appeal to my subconscious mind for help in improving my speed as a writer, sharpening my tennis game, and developing my social skills, as well as controlling my anxious reactions to business pressures. My proficiency with these creative visualization techniques was directly proportional to the frequency with which I practiced them. I also learned how to circumvent my resistance to change by experimenting with different types of suggestions, to entice my subconscious into cooperating in the problem-solving processes. The never-ending contest of willpower versus want, or "me versus me," has intrigued me ever since.

During this period, I also met Dr. Lawrence Beuret, whose medical practice included patients with psychosomatic (mind/body) disorders, such as claustrophobia, agoraphobia, post-traumatic stress disorder, and "irrational" fears that manifested as physical illnesses. He contracted me to write patient information brochures, case studies, and feature articles on his success with these unusual illnesses and disorders. As a result, I gained more insights into the fascinating subconscious, including why it produced "unacceptable behavior" (such as phobias) in the mistaken belief it was protecting a person from danger. Dr. Beuret also taught me more subconscious communication techniques for enlisting the subconscious mind to help a person "correct" the faulty belief system, and therefore help control or diminish the unwanted behavior.

As the doctor explained, the subconscious mind, in addition to being the protector of the "self," is the keeper of all memories. Every event, thought, feeling, and sensual perception a person experiences from conception to the present is dutifully recorded by the subconscious. These memories are stored and linked by the accompanying emotion of the moment and—this is important—cataloged by degrees of emotional impact. For example, if I eat an ice cream cone right now, it will reinforce and link emotionally with my now consciously forgotten memory of the first ice cream cone I tasted as a toddler, as well as with all the ice cream cone memories in between. This initial emotional memory is cataloged in the high impact area of my subconscious. I call it "high impact" for two reasons: First, it was recorded before my conscious mind developed, and second, it has been constantly reinforced through the years.

Because the conscious mind does not develop until around age seven, this initial memory of pure joy dominates many of my other joyful memories, because it is unadulterated by logical conscious thoughts, such as "Eating ice cream makes you fat." In addition, over the next 50 years of my life, I've reinforced the initial ice cream joy memory many times. Perhaps that's why I almost always feel an urge to run to the freezer for a pick-me-up after a bad day. Subconsciously speaking, over the years, an ice cream cone has come to mean more to me than a delicious frozen dairy product; it also brings back that feeling of joy.

Let's say my first ice cream cone experience happened on a sandy beach. The humidity was 80 percent, seagulls were calling in the distance, the scent of baby lotion filled the air, and, with each ice cream drip, my doting parents took turns wiping the ice cream residue off my chin. These seemingly insignificant details were emotionally linked and recorded as part of the initial ice cream memory event. Theoretically speaking, any of those accompanying details—for instance, the call of seagulls—is capable either of arousing my desire for an ice cream cone or inspiring a feeling of joy and contentment.

Meanwhile, the logical conscious mind (unaware of any of these subconscious factors) is baffled by my craving for an ice cream cone when I'm sitting on the beach or whenever I am discontented. In fact, I could tell myself that "ice cream makes me fat" until I am blue in the face, and still these logical words would have no power over my "illogical" emotional craving for an ice cream cone. These more recent conscious thoughts, however, do affect how I perceive an ice cream cone today. Never again will I totally experience an ice cream cone with the unabashed joy of a two-year-old. Instead, my later-life ice cream memories will be watered down emotionally because I'll be thinking "downer" thoughts such as "I'm cheating on my diet," "I should have ordered maple nut; I prefer it over chocolate," or "Darn, I dripped it on my blouse," and so forth. But all of these logical thoughts are still no match for the initial emotional experience. Even though my ever-controlling conscious mind is fooled into thinking it has the "whole ice cream story," it is wrong. And thus the craving continues.

After several years, my business relationship ended with the doctor and we lost contact, though I had heard he had switched the focus of his practice to treating attention disorders in young people. It never occurred to me to contact him for help with Eve's stroke condition, although (if I had thought about it) her rehabilitation needs did touch on areas of his expertise. Eve's aneurysm/strokes were certainly a mind-body disorder, she did have significant problems paying attention, and she suffered both short- and long-term memory loss.

In summary, I held these beliefs about the subconscious mind. The subconscious is Protector of the Self, Keeper of the Value System, and Librarian in charge of cataloging all conscious and subconscious memories. Looking back, I did not formally plan a subconscious rehabilitation strategy. Now I wish my approach had been more scientific, but then I was grasping for straws of hope.

As you will see, Eve's rehabilitation strategy evolved from day to day as I began to realize I was continually soliciting the subconscious Protector to assist me on safety and health issues, pleading with the subconscious Value Keeper to provide the missing spark of motivation so that Eve could rejoin life, and forever appealing to the Memory Librarian to help me go fishing for the links that would connect Eve's present with her now-forgotten emotional past.

Since subconscious communication is a two-way street, it is essential that my subconscious has a clear picture of my personal motives here.

In the 12-Step program, our primary motive for sponsoring is to maintain our sobriety, not to help someone else. Selfish as that may sound, it works to banish all those victim and martyr reactions we might have if a sponsee drinks again.

In Eve's case, I tell myself that her rehabilitation is important for my self-preservation because I don't want to be a caregiver for the rest of my life. I need to believe I'm doing meaningful rehabilitation work. Second, I tell myself that my rehabilitation role is important to my value system, because of our long-ago mutual promise to care for each other in case of illness. Third, if I can't help Eve reconnect with her emotions or her personality, I'll be facing the prospect of a deadly dull life together. It's imperative that I help Eve retrieve some aspects of her short- and long-term memories for our personal safety.

Last, but not least, I really need to teach Eve how to cook again—or
we may starve to death. Yessiree, I'm motivated in my corner.
Nowhere to go but up.

In essence, these suggestions to myself fulfill one of the criteria
for connecting with the subconscious: They are all emotion-based
appeals. But I know it's nearly impossible to keep that emotion level
high day after day. I will need to couch my appeals in an easy-to-
remember creative visualization that illustrates what I am trying to
accomplish and also keeps my enthusiasm level high.

Ah, how the subconscious mind loves pictures. Luckily, I am primarily a "visual" thinker. One picture that has been playing in my
mind since November features me shoveling snow from the paths in
Eve's brain to create new routes around the aneurysm-damaged
area: simple, satisfying, and a good pictorial metaphor for what I am
trying to do every day. Over time, I incorporate another visualization,
which I dub "fishing for Eve's memories and emotion strings." In
actuality, I've never been into fishing; I can't get past the worm.
Rather, I remember a childhood game I used to play. It involved
using a magnetized fishing pole to capture colorful little metal fish
cutouts. The game must have been great fun because the memory
keeps popping up every time I try to visualize Eve's broken memory
chain. Subconsciously speaking, the image and action are picture-
perfect for my plan to snag any "piece" of Eve's emotional memory
strings, in hopes of reeling in the whole big kahuna.

Next on the agenda is how will I prioritize all the areas that I
need to address with Eve and manage the house? Well, gosh, I could
ask my subconscious that one. As a career writer, I've often encoun-
tered that deadline-threatening curse known as "writer's block." All
successful writers have tricks to get around it. My favorite is "Sleep on
it." It's a simple process. Sometime before bed, I write a short outline
describing my writing assignment. Then, before I fall asleep, I ask my
subconscious to help me "think it through" during the night and
present a solution sometime the next morning. I also emphasize that
a "solution" is required for my survival on the job, which, of course,
is directly connected to my need for food, shelter, and clothing, as

well as various other things I hold dear. I cannot remember any time an earnest subconscious petition has gone unanswered.

Okay, that takes care of my side of the street. Now, what about Eve? As I see it, our success rests with how skillfully I can align my suggestions with Eve's lifelong belief system. These include:

- No matter what happens, Eve believes God will take care of her (in the style to which she has become accustomed).

- Eve is proud of her role as homemaker and chief cook throughout her 20-year marriage and the current household arrangement.

- Eve believes in the basic goodness of people. She lives the Golden Rule: Do unto others as you would have them do unto you.

- Eve's "religion" is a mix of Catholic teachings and 12-Step program Higher Power concepts. Her visualization of God is "the big A.A. sponsor in the sky."

- The product of a Polish culture, Eve believes that living on credit is a "sin," cleanliness is next to godliness, and your home is your castle.

- One of Eve's missions in life is to be available to help people in need, primarily aging relatives. She is proud of helping Donna develop as an artist and of her own support role as the "framing specialist."

- Eve believes "work" (as in earning a living) is a four-letter word.

- Eve's self-concept is that she is lazy when it comes to self-improvement issues. So she believes: If at first she doesn't succeed, maybe she'll think about trying the next time.

- Eve has always had a "flat" emotional response to life; she's always happy. She maintains that her happy-go-lucky, humorous approach to problems is the key to her emotional survival.

The final aspect of my subconscious rehabilitation plan is perhaps the most daunting: verbally communicating with dopey Eve. In two-way subconscious communication, it will help if I address Eve's various problems in everyday-speak and not in the technical terms and complicated explanations used by the professional medical community. I'll be more at ease telling myself and Eve what's going on and what I want in my words.

And for Eve's part? Well, she certainly is relaxed. But how to get Eve to focus? She is so heavily medicated and/or brain-damaged that she appears to have the attention span of a flitting bird most of the time.

I've noticed, however, that she takes more interest in what I say immediately after dinner. She seems to exhibit an "air of expectation" at that moment, similar to someone asking, "So, what's for dessert?" I also perceive that feeling after breakfast, as if the question is "What's on the agenda today?" Could be my wishful thinking, but it may also be my perception of Eve's lifetime habit of asking that question and expecting an answer. Anyway, it's a place to start.

I also recall a nurse at the nursing home telling me to deliver messages into Eve's left ear while maintaining left eye contact. The reason, she said, was that Eve's left side was stronger than the right, which was affected by the stroke. I incorporated this method into my "Eve approach" to deliver short "safety" messages to her. Those attempts seemed to be successful. In actuality, I had never tested it to see how long I could hold Eve's attention. I make a mental note to become more aware of her responses.

Communication is not a one-way street. I have noticed on numerous occasions that Eve communicates several other ways besides verbally. For instance, toward the end of her speech therapy sessions, Eve would begin yawning. The yawn didn't seem to indicate sleepiness so much as a physical attempt to take in more oxygen for her brain so that it could focus. If I suggested something that displeased her, she'd immediately look away and start playing with her earlobe, seemingly signaling that this conversation was over. And on more than one occasion she did the opposite of whatever was requested, unable to hide a distinctly mischievous smile, indicating she "knew" she was teasing and/or tormenting me. Yep, dear Eve was still as passive-aggressive as ever, especially around me.

My job, as I see it, is to couch my suggestions creatively so they're emotionally irresistible to Eve's subconscious. After 30 years in advertising, I shouldn't have too much of a problem with that. There are numerous techniques for communicating with the subconscious, including creative visualization, direct suggestion, body language, and reframing.

In the end, I opt for a watered-down version of creative visualization, which I call "storytelling" or reminiscing, to counter Eve's short attention span. Besides the brain destruction wrought by the bursting aneurysm and the effects of mind-numbing medications, I theorize (that is, I guess) that Eve's ability to focus is further diminished by a continuous high anxiety state of the brain. Well, why wouldn't the poor thing be anxious? It's been badly injured and every time it tries to function "normally," the signals are rerouted or blocked or otherwise sabotaged. I would bet it's also tired of trying hard to respond to therapist requests and my caregiver requests, too. That's a lot of stress for a poor little brain that's trying to heal.

Rewiring a brain is the stuff of which good science fiction is created. But when the choice is thinking that way or cohabitation with a crippled mind in the middle of nowhere, I'm ready to believe anything is possible just for a reason to wake up in the morning. At this moment, a favorite A.A. slogan comes to mind: "Act as if." Okay, I will "act as if" it's possible to entice the brain to make new circuits using direct subconscious suggestion and creative visualization. It certainly can't hurt Eve for me to try, and it'll give me an organized approach to dealing with all the surprises that brain-damage behavior presents during the day.

How do I know I can't hurt Eve? For the very same reason that the subconscious mind is the protector of Eve's value system and the harbor of her survival instinct. No matter what I suggest to her, if her subconscious doesn't believe it will enhance or ensure her survival, it will be rejected. I suppose a top-secret brainwashing program might be able to get around that, but that's way beyond my capabilities and certainly not my motivation. This approach should work best—and fastest—the closer I can align it with Eve's lifelong values, her inventory of memories, and her typical emotional reactions to everyday living.

# 15

# A Meeting of the Minds

If I intend to communicate with Eve's subconscious, perhaps I should shape up my own subconscious first.

It's in a sorry state. Between the stress effects and anxiety attacks, I've really let myself go. What's the payoff here?

Hmmm. I rather enjoy the image of myself as a martyr. It's a refreshing change from my usual self-centeredness. But really, how much fun is it without an audience? Eve hardly qualifies. Now is the time to get serious about taking care of myself. I can start by brushing up on my rusty relaxation methods, beginning with the tried-and-true progressive relaxation technique. While I am at it, I can use this opportunity to deliver a more formal message to my subconscious mind, asking it to relieve that overwhelmed feeling. Actually, I'm always asking it for some kind of help, but it will pay more attention to a formal request. I can pack more punch in a relaxed state, which is a rather rare occasion these days.

Beginning with a reminder to stay focused, I visualize sunbathing on a tropical beach, the surf rolling in, the sun on my back. Then I take three deep breaths and slowly count from one to ten, imagining the soothing warmth traveling from toe to head, stopping to relax various body parts along the way. When I arrive at "ten," I'm in a relaxed, daydream state, perfect for delivering my message to myself.

"Dear subconscious, please help me utilize your powers to relax and be more efficient through the day. Please show me how to relieve the stress. You are invited to join me in a brainstorming session following this exercise. Thank you." Counting backward from ten to one, I give myself the message to become more alert and energized.

Though a relaxed state helps in delivering a message, it's also imperative for the other half of the subconscious communication process: listening.

Years ago, when I was an advertising writer in the hectic, deadline-oriented ad agency environment, I practiced "instant" subconscious communications more proficiently. I signaled for its attention with a key word that triggered an immediate relaxed state and receptive environment for ideas.

Now I'm woefully out of practice, so I need to establish a two-way communications ritual, such as a brainstorming session. The blank sheet of paper in front of me is a not-too-subtle signal to the subconscious that it's time to talk and I'm listening.

Doodling helps, while I wait for ideas to flow. If nothing happens in the next 15 minutes, I'll divert my attention with a chore, then return to my brainstorming session in an hour.

Sometimes the subconscious can be a little ornery, especially if I keep interrupting it with worrisome conscious thoughts. If need be, I'll do another progressive relaxation exercise to show it that I'm listening.

Guess it's my lucky day. My subconscious seems eager to volunteer all sorts of different ways it can help me. The pen is flying across the pages.

First, the subconscious can prioritize my daily chores. Between caregiving, rehabilitation, homemaking, and bill paying, I've been wasting time trying to decide what to do next. If I just ask my subconscious for its help at night before falling asleep, it will prioritize the next day's tasks while I dream. When I awaken, the day's duties will magically line up in my mind in order of importance. Experience has taught me that somehow I'll automatically know how much time to devote to each task.

Here comes another idea. My subconscious suggests that I'm worrying way too much about the bills. Relax; take things one month at a time. This month, we're okay. But what about that pile of outrageous medical bills and those incomprehensible insurance statements? Instead of reading a magazine, I could write letters while waiting for Eve at the rehab center. Flag the bills that need attention, then trust that the subconscious will find the right words to ask for explanations, concessions, or manageable payment plans or to dispute charges without ruffling anyone's feathers. And watch that temper of yours, it warns me.

How about the cloud of financial doom hanging over our heads? I don't know whether to put the house on the market, or look for a job and pay someone to watch Eve, or find some way to earn money at home. As I doodle, I can hear a little voice telling me to table the house and job issues until May. By then, Eve will be finished with outpatient rehabilitation and the job market will open up as the tourism season begins. The real estate market will follow soon after. It does no good to worry until then. Put the whole sorry mess on hold.

Now my subconscious mind is bugging me with an annoying thought. Try as I might, I can't push it away. Just because I've tabled the house and job issues until spring doesn't mean I can't institute cost-cutting measures now. Reluctantly, I bite the bullet, making a note to discontinue our second phone line for the computer. Happy now? As time goes on, I'm sure my subconscious will spit out all sorts of ways to save money. Now, don't pout, I admonish myself. Remember how challenging being poor was in your early days of sobriety. At least you weren't bored. That's when you rediscovered the treasures awaiting you at the public library. Shelf upon shelf of books, videos, and CDs, and everything was free. Okay. I grudgingly thank my subconscious for the idea and make a note to visit the library this week.

Switching to the homemaking front, there's the immediate problem of planning and cooking easy, nutritious dinners. My limited repertoire of meals has been further reduced by Eve's inability to consistently chew and swallow correctly. I'd avoid the kitchen completely if there were an inexpensive fast-food option nearby. But alas, northern Door County prides itself on not allowing fast-food chains. The concept of "quaint" is wearing a little thin these days.

While Eve was institutionalized, I happily lost my appetite and a few pounds. But now that Eve is home, I'm getting hungry. Guess I better start reading Eve's cookbooks. But wait, I have a better idea. Oh, thank you, subconscious. I write a note to call Cass. She said she wants to help. She's a gourmet cook. She'll know recipes that match my skill level. Maybe she can email them and save me time from wracking my brain, thumbing through cookbooks for ideas.

Back to doodling. My mind is whirling; nothing's clear. I look down at the doodles. Letters and shapes. Hmmm, looks like a mini-billboard. That triggers an idea. Billboards, the essence of advertising science and art, the only format with explicit rules: a stunning visual and a simple, motivating slogan, never more than ten words.

That's it! I can use billboards to remind myself to stay calm, to motivate me through the day, and, perhaps, to deliver simple messages to Eve. I've got a clean sheet of paper. Let's try one or two.

Let's start with "calm." So what calms me? The lake, of course. A few squiggles—lake waves! Hmmm. A triangle for a sailboat. Doesn't matter if nobody else recognizes what I've drawn; I know what it represents. And my slogan? "Let go, let God." Ah! There—a billboard! I'll tape that one to the refrigerator.

Now I need one for Eve. Where the heck is she? Oh, yeah, watching golf on TV. "Hey, Eve, mute it! I'm going to create a billboard for you. How about that? Let's see, what shall I draw? How about two smiley faces? We'll put curly hair on this one, that's me. We'll put chic straight hair on this one—wait, I've got to get the part that's standing straight up—that's SO you.

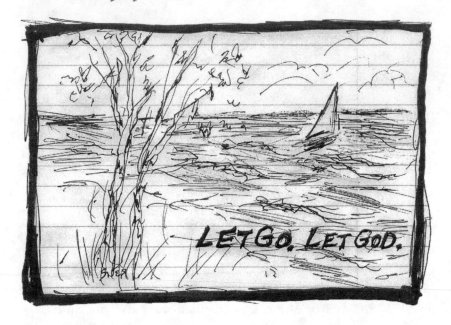

"And we're going to say—I want you to pay attention here, Eve—listen and believe: 'We will get better together.' How about if I tape this to the bathroom mirror?"

"Uh-huh."

"Alright, you can go back to your golf. I've got to see if there's anything else to brainstorm."

Back at the dining room table, I doodle, doodle. Minutes pass. Uh-oh. As quickly as they came, the ideas stop coming. Into the vacuum of my mind marches one big conscious question: This is all fine, but how do I rehabilitate Eve?

What a downer. Slowly I start doodling again, unsure if my subconscious even has a clue on how to answer that question. Stop it. Now I'm consciously thinking instead of receiving ideas. Okay, I'll stop—but the question remains. Why am I fighting to find a way to help Eve, when everyone says there's nothing I can do? Time will heal Eve, not you. Maybe I should just surrender, pick up my marbles, and go home. Resign myself to the life of a helpless caregiver, watching Eve flounder while I pray for a miracle to heal her damaged brain. Excuse me, but if time is the healer, and there's nothing

I can do, why is the insurance company paying NEW thousands of dollars? To do what? Wait for time to do its thing?

No, I'm not giving up yet. Come on, subconscious. Give me a few more minutes of brainstorming on this problem. If nothing comes, I'll end the session. As I doodle, my thoughts flit back to this morning, when I reaffirmed my commitment to use the concepts from the 12-step program. Yeah, so? Is there a message here, subconscious? Okay, I'll go with it. First, I admitted powerlessness and that I believed a Higher Power could help. I know it's a program of action and that I always turn over the results to the care of a power greater than myself. Hmmm, just like my billboard: "Let go, let God." But I still don't see how the program can help me with Eve.

That triggers another memory, this time from my beginner days in A.A. Like many of the uninitiated, I objected to the concept of powerlessness or relying on a Higher Power on the grounds that "I had been there, done that." Hadn't I prayed for years, asking God to please stop my drinking? It didn't work then; why should it now? My always-patient sponsor explained that belief in a Higher Power required positive action on my part to demonstrate that belief to myself. Even an alternative routine action, such as mopping a floor, would have prevented me from picking up a drink.

"What does mopping a floor have to do with drinking? I don't get it," I told my sponsor.

With a sigh, she suggested that maybe I should simply believe that she believes the program works . . . and, by the way, go mop a floor.

Doesn't that sound crazy? Sure, it does. But the suggestion came from a woman who was happily sober . . . and I, with all my "sane, logical" thinking was still stuck on Step One. "Okay," I reluctantly surrendered. "I'll believe that you believe. Now what do I do?"

"Mop the floor, then go to a meeting," she suggested.

"Okay, then what?"

"Keep calling for more direction one day at a time. And by the way," she added, "congratulations, you're finally working the program."

"How's that?" I asked.

"By believing that taking this action will help you."

"Huh? I don't get it."

"Never mind. You don't have to understand what you're doing right now."

That was worth a chuckle. But, hey, I'm wasting time reminiscing. Obviously, there's no way I can use the 12 Steps to rehabilitate Eve physically, mentally, or emotionally. Or is there? Was there a message in that memory?

Perhaps the answer isn't in the Steps, per se. Maybe it's in the method of teaching the Steps. It's not easy teaching anything to despairing A.A. beginners with soggy brains. In my case, it took me several months before I could add two and two again. During that time, I relied on my sponsor for daily direction. "Today, you'll mop the kitchen floor; do one load of laundry; be sure to eat lunch; take a shower; apply for one job, doing anything; eat dinner; and I'll pick you up tonight for a meeting."

How low can one go? Wasn't it humiliating? Not for someone as sick as I was. Besides, in A.A. we're taught no matter how awful our experience was, we can use it to help someone else. The role of the sponsor evolved out of the A.A. program's Twelfth Step. Having been healed, we should share our experience, strength, and hope with other beginners. The process of giving away the wisdom we gained from our experience allows us to keep it for ourselves.

In order to help me, my sponsor revisited her own bottom, when she, too, was a brain-damaged neophyte in A.A. needing similar direction to make it through the day. Those of us who have visited the bottom of alcoholism know that the steps won't "take" until the brain has a chance to repair the damage wrought by alcohol. That doesn't mean, however, that the low-bottom beginners sit and twiddle their thumbs, waiting to heal. They "act as if" they get it, by attending A.A. meetings. Is there a way I can connect this experience with my current caregiving situation? I wonder.

But first, time for a break. Eve wants lunch. I artistically plop some yogurt, fruit, and cottage cheese on a plate. Yum. I can tell by Eve's lack of enthusiasm that this woman wants ham and Swiss on rye. Feeding her real food would mean supervising every little bite she takes, making sure she chews, swallows, then follows each bite with a sip of water. B-o-r-i-n-g.

As Eve pushes away the unfinished plate of cottage cheese, I realize I'll have to make that decision soon. If she doesn't eat enough to meet her caloric-consumption requirements, then meals will have to be supplemented with an expensive high-calorie drink, sipped through a straw or, heaven forbid, poured into the feeding tube. Yuck. The thought of cleaning that feeding tube more than once a day makes me shudder. I decide watching her eat isn't so bad, after all.

"Okay, Eve, if you'll just eat mush for one more week, I promise you can graduate to real food next Saturday. Now finish that cottage cheese." Afterward, I give her an art book to thumb through while I take a bathroom break, bringing Eve's billboard with me. Hmmm, we'll get better together. Wonder where that came from?

Back to my dining room table doodles. My revitalized subconscious continues to pursue the A.A. sponsor train of thought. How can this apply?

There must be a huge difference between the amount of brain damage inflicted by alcoholism and the chaos created by a bursting brain aneurysm and strokes. But A.A. trains us to look for the similarities in our experience and not focus on the differences. I consider Eve at face value, as if we met at an A.A. meeting. She's dopey, unable to focus her attention, off-balance; she's unable to perform simple tasks, can't hold a thought, doesn't communicate intelligently, doesn't seem to feel her emotions. Doesn't that sound just like me when I came into the A.A. program? Anyway, Eve is on Zoloft for depression and Ritalin for attention-deficit problems. In those pre-Prozac days of my early sobriety, my depression and anxiety disorders went untreated. Does that level the playing field a little? At the very least, I know what it's like to try to function in a fog, and the frustration of not being able to communicate. Perhaps my imagination and my experience with others can make up for the rest of the difference between our brain-damage experiences.

I notice Eve is staring at me, a meaningless smile on her face.

"You want something?" I ask. She shakes her head. "Talk," I command, out of frustration. "Say yes or no."

"No," she obliges.

"Please, God," I pray, "I don't want to create a self-cleaning, self-feeding robot. Please, help me bring back the old Eve."

Looking down at my notes, I argue with myself. Sponsoring Eve à la A.A. is really a stretch, but . . . oh heck. Go for it. It's time to share my plan with her.

"Eve, please pay attention. This may sound crazy, but I've decided to sponsor you into brain recovery. It'll be like A.A., only different. You didn't know me in the beginning, but I was brain-damaged and dopey, too. Maybe not as bad as you, but close enough for me. Anyway, I'm all you have right now. If I got better, then you can, too. You do want to get well, don't you?"

Eve nods.

"So first admit that you're powerless to do it yourself. If you accept that, then the next step is to put your trust in me, as your caregiver-sponsor, and my directions for rehabilitation, based on my experience. Then you'll proceed one task at a time to recover your brain."

Eve stares at me blankly.

"Okay, that went well. You have no idea what I'm talking about, do you? Hmmm. It is a 'we' program. Maybe I can accept your powerlessness over your brain damage for you. Then we can both 'act as if' this plan is going to work. I'll keep my expectations low, but there'll be no more namby-pamby caregiving. This is a program of action. You'll do the things you don't want to do. At least, I expect you to try. Trying counts. But you'll accept the consequences of your actions. I believe that somewhere inside you the 'old Eve' still has a say. That's who I'll be talking to, I hope."

Eve nods again.

"Talk," I command.

"Yes," Eve says, almost assertively.

"Good. Now, maybe we can get better together." My words stun me. So that's what I was saying to myself: Sponsor Eve. That's worth a celebration. "Come on, Eve. Let's have some ice cream."

After our treat, I put aside my brainstorming for the weekend. I can hear three loads of laundry calling me without the aid of my subconscious. Anyway, my subconscious has enough tasks for the week. I'll resume the tête-à-tête with my mind next Saturday. I hope my subconscious will have figured out our next step by then.

The following Thursday, Valentine's Day, is Eve's first social outing. I'm treating her to dinner at our favorite Swedish restaurant in Sister Bay, a quaint Door County tourist town 20 minutes away. The restaurant's specialty, Swedish meatballs, is one of Eve's favorites. That's good, because they're relatively easy to cut and chew and, best of all, affordable.

Maybe we'll look like an odd couple on the lovers' holiday. But, heck, just because there's no man in my life, or Eve's, doesn't mean we should deny ourselves a midwinter holiday celebration.

As soon as we arrive at the restaurant, I hurry Eve into the restroom. Perhaps I'm overreacting to Eve's continence issue, but I don't want to spoil the festivities worrying about an accident. I even went so far as to pack a complete change of clothes for her. At least I left them in the car. Since Eve just went to the bathroom 20 minutes ago, the exercise is fruitless. Good thing I never had to toilet-train a toddler. I would've ended up in the funny farm.

I guide Eve into the dining room, avoiding wayward chairs and bustling waitresses. Eve manages to seat herself without falling over. Oblivious to my overconcern for Eve, the waitress hands us the menus and promises to return to take our orders. Eve pipes up that she wants a steak.

"If you order a steak," I threaten, "I'll have to cut it up into tiny pieces for you. Everyone will look at us. Do you want that?"

Disappointed, Eve shakes her head.

"Besides, it costs too much," I whisper. "Anyway, this is your chance to have Swedish meatballs. You can get a steak anywhere. I'll even let you try cutting your own meatballs. How about that?" I wince at my boldness, as the image of a wayward meatball flying across the room dances through my mind.

Eve smiles and nods.

The waitress reappears to take our orders. "Two Swedish meatball dinners and iced teas," I say, purposely passing up the chance to let Eve practice ordering her own meal. I'd bet my bottom dollar she has already forgotten our conversation and would order that steak. The waitress disappears and I notice Eve looking longingly at a romantic couple, enjoying their dinner a few tables away.

"What's the matter," I ask. "Do you miss your husband, Richard?"

Eve shakes her head. "No, I was wondering if you wanted to split a bottle of wine."

"Oh, you betcha. Best idea you've had in years. Only one problem, Eve. I don't want a half a bottle of wine; I want a whole bottle, all for myself, and one to go. Have you forgotten we're members of that elite club known as A.A.?" I resist the urge to throttle her neck. "Please don't tempt me in my state of mind. Now, repeat after me," I whisper, "I am a recovering alcoholic. Drinking is not an option."

As she mumbles the phrase, I see a flicker of awareness in her eyes. "I'm sorry. I forgot," she adds. "Thank you for reminding me. Iced tea is fine."

As we wait for dinner, I feel a little shaky. Damn, I'm "booze-fighting," trying to will away the thought that nobody will know or care if I relapse in rural Wisconsin. Alas, willpower never helps in these situations. Finally, my 13 years of recovery comes to my rescue. Silently, I admit my powerlessness over the thought of drinking. But just because I have the thought doesn't mean I should act on it by actually ordering a bottle of wine. There. Thank you, God. Like magic, my craving disappears.

By the time the waitress serves us, I'm ready to enjoy dinner and devote my attention to helping Eve manage her meatballs. As I had hoped, the dinner is the highlight of our weary week.

Saturday afternoon, it's time for another brainstorming session with my subconscious. Eve has finished consuming her "first" ham and Swiss on rye sandwich, thankfully without incident. She's in the bathroom now. We haven't had a daytime incontinence accident for several days, primarily because I take her to the bathroom every two hours.

Why hasn't Eve called me to retrieve her from the bathroom? She's been quiet way too long. I hurry in. Eve's on the toilet—reading. Somehow, the brain aneurysm missed the clump of neurons associated with that old habit. Wonders never cease. As we walk down the hallway, I survey the results of our morning dual shower/shampoo/blow-dry session. Her short, straight, silvery "do" is flying in all directions. Obviously, I'm not much of a hairstylist. My own hair feels sticky with shampoo residue, two weeks' worth. I still haven't mastered cleaning myself and keeping an eye on towel-wrapped Eve. Now she's getting bolder. Despite my pleading, she won't wait for me to finish my shower. Instead, she attempts to dry herself, including her toes. Watching Eve try to balance herself is an unnerving experience—sort of like watching a clown perform a high-wire act. No wonder there's still soap in my hair.

I direct Eve into the living room and her favorite comfy leather chair, now protected by a disposable bed pad. I wrap an afghan around her shoulders, serve her a cup of tea, and flip on the TV.

"Ah, that's what I'm looking for. Here, Eve, you can watch this golf tournament. Mentally, practice your strokes. See if you can beat the pros. I'll be at the table, if you want anything."

Looking out the patio doors, I notice that the sky has a warm robin's egg blue tint to it. Looks like spring to me! I can even see water holes in the harbor ice. Whoopee! Everything's melting.

Okay, back to work. After reviewing my notes from last week's session, I'm feeling more confident. True, I'm stretching the concept of sponsoring beyond the traditional 12-Step approach by imagining I'm powerless along with Eve. But don't I try to empathize with every beginner I sponsor?

Moving along, I recall my sponsor's Step 2 sermon. "Unless you acknowledge that you're sick, how can you possibly get well?" This really applies now. Since Eve isn't aware of her disabilities, I'll acknowledge them for her. I realize I've been looking at her disabilities piecemeal. Perhaps I should write an all-inclusive list so we have a starting point. I divide her disabilities into three categories, minus the mumbo-jumbo medical terminology the professionals use.

Physically—Eve can't walk in a straight line; she doesn't turn her head or swing her arms while walking. She loses her balance rising from a chair. Her shoulder appears to be frozen by stroke. Raising her arm over her head is uncomfortable, if not painful. She favors using her left hand; her right is weakened by the stroke. She's incontinent, often unaware of any bodily signals to eliminate. She doesn't even know when it's time to blow her nose or clear her throat. She shivers all the time, but won't try to warm herself. Her chewing-swallowing mechanism is minimally functioning.

Mentally—Eve is oblivious to personal safety issues. Though she manages the toilet routine, she resists bathing. She doesn't like the "feel" of water on her head in the shower. She appears to use little judgment in choosing her clothes, even when given a limited choice. She doesn't initiate any task, even the ones she can accomplish, such as fixing a bowl of cereal. Her long-term memory is spotty. Her short-term memory is a disaster. She can't recall a phone conversation after hanging up the phone. She's often confused. She confabulates ("lies") to help her make sense of disparities between past memories and present circumstances. For instance, she tells me to take the dogs for a walk when she really means feed the cats. Or she says that her late husband stopped by when it was the handyman. She usually doesn't speak unless spoken to. Most of her responses are a word or a phrase, rarely more than one sentence.

Emotionally—alas, poor Eve has been robbed of her ability to feel anything other than mild happiness or disappointment. Though I'm grateful she doesn't exhibit the angry or crying behavior of many stroke victims, her inappropriate smiling is driving me nuts. It seems she recognizes her friends, but she reacts to all of us in the same unenthusiastic manner.

Wow, that's quite a list, and I'll bet I missed some things. . . . Hey, what was that noise? I quickly check Eve. She's okay. I hear it again. Oh, it's just the ice cracking in the harbor. Maybe it's a sign? Maybe I'm on the verge of a breakthrough? Oh, shut up and get back to work.

# A Meeting of the Minds

All week long a new thought has been bugging me. Though I'm thrilled about the attention Eve's therapists lavish on her, something's been bothering me about the therapy method. It's so function oriented. Not just at NEW, but in Chicago, too. I'm not sure what I would or could do to change it, but it all seems so fruitless. Who cares if Eve can move her arm better when there's no "life" in her mirthless smile and vacant stare? How will handgrip exercises ever bring back the old Eve?

There is one session that brings a light to Eve's eyes. It's called "executive skills." The administrator is allowing Eve to participate, although it's beyond her current capabilities. The class focuses on summarizing and prioritizing lists of information. The patients also practice making decisions. Despite her task initiation and comprehension difficulties, Eve still tries to rise to the challenge. I know the other therapies try to increase her skill level, but the "game" doesn't appeal to Eve. I can almost hear her saying, "This is really stupid" or "What's the point?" How can I use this to help build my therapy program? I wonder.

Apparently, my subconscious doesn't know the answer because I'm not receiving any ideas. Perhaps inspired by my instruction to Eve to practice her golf strokes, however, I have an irresistible urge to create another billboard. On a fresh piece of paper I quickly draw a stick figure swinging a golf club. My slogan is simply: "Act as if." There. Done. Now I feel a little bit better. Another billboard for the refrigerator.

Okay, that's enough for today. But before I quit, I want to impress my subconscious with the long list of Eve's disabilities before I'm too tired to relax and focus. I repeat the progressive relaxation routine, then deliver my message.

"Dear subconscious, I'm asking your help in rehabilitating Eve. (I read aloud the list of disabilities.) This is our starting point. Our goal is to bring back the old Eve. How do I motivate her to rise to the challenge? I'm asking for your help. Thank you." Then I count backward.

Rats. I don't feel revitalized at all. Maybe I should say a little prayer.

"Dear God, please let me see what I have to see, hear what I have to hear, say what I have to say, and do what I have to do, in order to do Your will."

I don't want to confuse God's power with that of my subconscious mind's power. For now, I'll limit the subconscious mind's tasks to providing strategies for Eve. My prayers to God will be for my own sanity, serenity, and acceptance of His will. Oh, who am I kidding? Of course, dear God, a miracle or two for Eve would be much appreciated.

The next morning, I awaken in a foul mood. Rats, it's snowing again. Yesterday's above-average temperatures had melted most of the backyard snow, revealing grass and other faded memories of our yard. The finches were chirping, or maybe those were chickadees. Anyway, I thought spring was just around the corner. That says a lot about my state of mind. It's mid-February in Door County, Wisconsin. What did I expect?

Darn. I'm not doing well at all. Just as I was relearning how to relax, I break my self-imposed rule of "no expectations." Plug one hole; spring a leak in another. Of course, if I just had a little more faith, I wouldn't have to worry about individual "leaks."

What's the matter with me, anyway? Didn't I conceive a nifty plan yesterday to heal Eve? Why don't I just relax and see how my plan unfolds?

"What plan?" I grumble to myself. All I know is what's wrong with Eve and that I want to bring her back. I have no idea how to get from here to there. There are hundreds of "holes" in Eve's mind. It'll take years to plug them all.

Wait a second. Plugging holes. Does that mean something? Darned if I know. If my subconscious is trying to teach a lesson here, it better clobber me over the head because I seem to be missing the point.

Meanwhile, first things first. I hurry Eve through her morning routine. As I watch her happily munching a bowl of Cheerios, I am momentarily mesmerized by those floating O's. I wonder: Are their little holes "plugged" by milk, or are they springing leaks? Depends on how you look at it, I guess. Perhaps my subconscious is trying to tell me not to worry about plugging holes. Just pour the milk and it will fill the holes. If a dry Cheerio pops up, just push it down. Ignore Eve's function-by-function rehab program. Approach the problem holistically. Create an imagined environment that Eve is already well. Act as if it's a fact. Slowly, but surely, it will seep into her brain holes.

I recall my last meeting with the neurosurgeon. He had cautioned me that Eve's recovery from here on was more a matter of time than rehabilitation efforts. "Wait and see what time does for her over the next 18 months."

"Excuse me, Doctor, but didn't you say there's only a two-year window for any major improvements? If I don't do anything for 18 months, and time doesn't cooperate by healing Eve, then what?"

The surgeon shrugged his shoulders. "You will have to wait and see."

Isn't that ridiculous? I've seen what happens if I allow time, alone, to heal a wound. I've got an ugly scar on my leg to show for it.

On the other hand, "time" is the closest thing to my idea of a holistic rehabilitation program for Eve. Maybe the doctor's right, or maybe he's just washing his hands of the problem, but I'm not sitting around waiting for "time" to do its thing.

Keep it simple, I remind myself. Alrighty, I will. I fetch Eve, who's been watching part two of the golf tournament. "This will only take a couple of minutes," I promise. "I'm going to read what's wrong with you to your subconscious, and then I'll ask it to heal you. Here, sit at the table. This is going to be simple, easy, and fun."

Eve looks appropriately bewildered.

"Okay, let's take three deep breaths." I eliminate the counting process. Eve is so dopey she doesn't need to relax deeply. Anyway, I don't know how long I can hold her attention. Next I read aloud my list of Eve's disabilities. Then I totally surprise myself with a new subconscious suggestion. "Please pay attention, subconscious minds. Both Eve and I need your help to plug the holes in her mind. We don't know how to do that; we don't even know what or where they are. But we trust that you do. We are going to act as if both of our subconscious minds want Eve to survive. I need your help to help her get well. Please help me be hypervigilant to any way I can help you reinforce your efforts or messages to Eve. Thank you." I count backward from ten to one, quickly say my prayer, then take Eve back to the TV golf tournament.

Wow, I feel relaxed, almost confident. Now I can turn the whole mess of how to proceed over to the care of my subconscious. My Higher Power can keep me sane in the process. Oh yes, I trust my Higher Power will help my subconscious whenever it gets stuck. Once upon a time, my Higher Power saved my life. So did my subconscious. I'll trust they can do it again. Yep. All I have to do is "act as if" this is going to work and then do the next right thing, which is . . . fix a bowl of ice cream.

"Hey, Eve, want some Chocolate Fudge Swirl?"

# 16

# A Program of Action

Last night, as I was drifting off to dreamland, I petitioned my subconscious for help in prioritizing the next day. I also asked it to help me stay calm, so that I might more readily recognize rehabilitation opportunities for Eve.

When I awoke this morning, however, I didn't feel that much different. I guess that's to be expected, since I am out of practice in following a relaxation routine. Yep, after the last few months of fervently practicing fear and anxiety, I just have to accept that it'll take a little time to replace those feelings with serenity—and courage.

So now I'm heading out to the backyard bluff to enlist some aid from my Higher Power in developing patience with myself. Before me is another dazzling "Door" morn—complete with winter sunrise, churning whitecaps, and bobbing ice blocks in the lake. Exhilarated yet calmed by the constancy of the lake waves, I ask my Higher Power for help with the new day. Then I recite my favorite prayer of Saint

Teresa: "Let nothing disturb thee. Let nothing dismay thee. All things pass. God never changes. Patience attains all that it strives for. He who has God finds he lacks nothing. God alone suffices." Slowly, but surely, I gain confidence in my plan to proceed through the day with patience for me and no expectations for rehabilitation results from Eve.

Maybe it's my yearning for a sign of spring that creates the visualization that is bouncing around in my brain. Nothing beats a good metaphor for helping me sort out the confusion about how to live everyday life. For example, there are things about my current predicament with Eve that remind me of one of my youthful pastimes. On any given summer's evening I might take a stroll to the neighborhood park. Usually, there was a Peanut League baseball game under way on one of the diamonds. I'd find a seat in the bleachers, amongst all those doting parents of peanut leaguers, and watch them watch their little tykes run around the diamond paying no attention to the baseball coach or their parents—the kids were just having fun.

It always amused me when a group of big adult "coaches" got together for a serious conference at first base, then whispered a base-running strategy to the seven-year-old who was too distracted to listen. Inevitably, the kid met his demise at second base, which caused more emotional reaction among the adults in the bleachers than among the kids.

Pity the poor parents who expected different results. How disappointing for them to invest such strong emotions in the outcome of the game when the team's talent potential was unknown and the skill level virtually undeveloped. Obviously, I had no emotional investment in the game's outcome, so I could just sit back and enjoy the show.

The rare home run and fly ball catches were rewards in themselves. The most memorable moments for me, however, were when some kindly coach gently corrected a mistake and tried to restore a little player's confidence to go back out and try again.

I'm sure that compassionate coach went home refreshed, untouched by expectations of winning or losing a game. In the end, he had done what every good kids' coach should do: light the fire of enthusiasm for playing the game, regardless of the outcome.

Not a bad visualization for me with Eve: Create an expectation-free environment that encourages "right action" and gently corrects mistakes as they happen. But we can never let "failure" keep us from going up to bat again . . . and again. We just have to keep playing the game.

Back inside the house, our day is beginning with a flurry—of snow, that is. All showered and toasty-warm in her terry-cloth robe, Eve is amusing herself by watching the gigantic flakes of snow float languorously in and out of the border of our picture-frame view of the lake. When I enter the room, she looks up at me expectantly.

"Hey, Eve, want to take a walk to the post office with me? Come on, let's get dressed."

We retreat to the bedroom where, as usual, I set out her sweatshirt, sweatpants, and socks for the day. I've taken particular pride in this portion of our daily routine. It's one of the few caregiving tasks I handle with any sense of confidence. But today I'm going to shake things up for both of us. As Eve stands at attention, waiting for me to undress/dress her, I announce, "Today, you will dress yourself."

My words shock me. Eve blinks in disbelief. What happened to Donna the caregiver?

"This is part of your rehabilitation program now," I tell her with all the tough love I can muster. "Take off your robe. Come on, get dressed."

Eve dutifully doffs her robe and nightgown, then sits down on the edge of the bed, shivering. I toss her the pants. "You've done this part a couple of times. Go ahead; tag in the back."

Eve struggles at first, eventually stands up, pulling up her pants, alternately swaying and regaining balance. "Good," I say. "Next, socks." She plops back down on the bed. She's grunting and groaning, but I keep warning her to get the heel and toe right or she'll have to start over. I feel like such a meanie, but too bad for me.

"Okay. Want to get warm? Here's your sweatshirt." (Thankfully, Eve's not "required" to wear a bra.)

Interesting. Eve checks the tag placement before I have a chance to say anything. Next she struggles to pull it over her head and partially place her arm in a sleeve. Apparently, her "frozen" shoulder is not cooperating.

"I can't," a muffled whine emanates from the folds of cloth. "My shoulder."

"Does it hurt, or is it just uncomfortable?" The mound of cloth nods. I'm sure she has lifted that arm before when I dressed her. I decide to go for it.

"Okay, Eve. I understand that you think your shoulder won't cooperate. But I believe you can put on that shirt. Start over, if you must."

"I can't get it off," comes the muffled reply.

"Yes, you can. Take all day, if you must." B-O-R-I-N-G.

*Voilà*—all of a sudden, the shirt is off. Inside out, but off.

"Okay, fix your shirt and we'll come up with a strategy." I can see that no matter what we do she'll have to raise that arm. I decide to take a pseudo-helpful approach, acting as if I've just thought of an easy way to do this.

"Okay, Eve. Here's what you do. Put the right arm in first, and then just go from there. That'll work." I turn away to hide my wincing.

Five minutes later, the shirt is on and Eve is panting. Twenty minutes altogether, including time-outs for whining. Can I do this every day, I wonder? "I don't know," a little voice in my head replies, "but you just might have to do your days in 20-minute segments. You're not a caregiver any more, and rehabilitation takes time."

Our next step is the coat wardrobe closet. "Pick a jacket, Eve, a winter one. That one doesn't have a hood, Eve. You won't be warm enough." Eve shrugs. "Okay, do it your way. Here, pick out a hat and mittens, and let's go."

Stepping outside, Eve begins shivering. "Want to go change your coat? No? Stubborn. Okay, you'll warm up walking. Now, I'm not going to hang on to you as we walk down this driveway. You can grab me if you lose your balance." (Of course, I'm ready to grab her if she does, but she doesn't know that.) "Watch out for ice and potholes. Watch where you're going."

Eve immediately stumbles, but I catch her. Testing me? "Watch out, keep your eyes on the ground. I'm staying behind you." She robotically zigzags down the drive, sort of like a drunk. "Stop at the curb," I call after her.

She does, and now it's time to impart another lesson. "Pay attention, Eve. This highway can be very dangerous, especially when the tourists come to town." Right now there isn't a car in sight. "Okay, repeat after me. I stop, I turn my head—first, I look left, then look right, then left again, and cross." We repeat my singsong chant until Eve's singing it solo. "You go first, Eve." Mission accomplished.

"Now we've got a choice, Eve. We can stay safe on the sidewalk and take the long way around. Or we can be adventurous and cut across this really bumpy empty lot, the way you always liked to go. Your choice."

"Cut across," she responds.

Okay, this will be an adventure. Probably because of her frozen shoulder, Eve doesn't swing her arms at all while walking. Keeping her balance might be a trick without that arm movement on the uneven terrain. I watch her take a few steps and teeter on top of a little snow mound.

"Whoa, Eve. Come here; give me your hand. We're going to swing arms while we march over the trail. Come on, we'll sing and swing. 'Over hill, over dale, as we hit the dusty trail . . . '"

Eve is giggling, concentrating on the arm swing and her singing. Consequently, she's not paying attention to overcorrecting for balance. Her subconscious is doing that for her. Pretty nifty trick. We virtually stride up to the steps of the post office.

"After you, my dear," I say. "I'll be right behind. Step right up and go inside. It's warm in there." At the top, Eve pauses to hold the door open for me. Nice touch. "So, Eve, do you remember your P.O. box number?"

Her blank stare tells me no. "Okay, 640. Can you find it?" Wow, she heads right to it. "Now, let's buy some stamps. Here's $10. You do it." I nod in the direction of the main room, and Eve swaggers—er, staggers—up to the front desk.

"Stamps, please," she says.

The clerk nods and smiles. It's not our regular postmaster.

Darn, I wanted to make some small talk, encourage some gossip. I try anyway. "Eve here has finally come home from the hospital."

The clerk nods and smiles a bit apprehensively. Obviously, he knows that. News has traveled around our tiny town. I presume he doesn't know much about brain aneurysms. He's acting as if Eve will bite him.

As the transaction ends, he cheerfully says, "Welcome back, Eve. Here's your change."

Eve smiles back. Good for her. Then she actually appears to count the change.

"Good for you, Eve," I tell her as we exit. "Today you picked up the mail and bought stamps. Congratulations. That's wonderful progress." Eve beams. "Now, let's head on back. We'll see if you can remember the words to the caisson song—and keep swinging those arms." By golly, she does.

Late that afternoon, a couple of Eve's friends telephone. Each time, I answer and tell Eve who it is. One is a second cousin from Chicago; the other is Eve's good friend, vivacious Penny. In both instances, I listen to Eve's side of the short conversations. To my dismay, she delivers a series of yes and no responses in the same flat voice. When I ask her, after she hangs up, to whom she talked, she replies, "A friend."

Geez, if jocular Penny can't elicit a more enthusiastic response, I don't know who can. I need people to keep calling to break up Eve's days (and mine). But now I begin to worry that it will only be a matter of time before the telephoners get bored or frustrated with Eve's monotone "conversation."

"You'll have to munch on that one," I instruct my subconscious, as I start dinner. Tonight's gourmet treat is blue-cheese burgers, fries, salad, and—ta-dah—chocolate almond ice cream. It's a pity to waste such a good dessert without using it as a reward for something. What's to reward? Not much has happened this afternoon and I don't actively try to rehab Eve after dinner. I'm usually too tired.

Wait a second. Cass will be phoning around seven o'clock. It's almost a ritual. Thank you, God, for Cass's calls and, more than that, her sense of humor. She's always poking fun at my all-too-serious approach to caregiving. Anyway, tonight I can ask to talk to Cass first. Maybe she can generate the enthusiasm I would like to reward.

Back to the task at hand. There are tomatoes to slice and onions to dice, and I've got to pay attention. I'm not a natural at veggie preparation. I could easily slice or dice a finger, instead.

"Come and get it," I call out to Eve, who's dozing in an easy chair. The evening news has lulled her to dreamland. It seems like 9/11 has been in the headlines forever. Funny how quickly my own personal "10/11" crisis wiped out my obsession with national news. Half-asleep, Eve responds to my call and begins to rise from the chair. Uh-oh, I can see she's off-balance. Dropping a fork, I run in and rescue her from disaster. "Please, Eve, think about what you're doing before you jump up. Count to three first, or something."

Hmmm. Burgers are pretty good. Perfect medium rare. I mentally pat myself on the back. "Slow down, Eve. Not such big bites. Chew three times, and then sip some water. Please, take it slow; you're relearning how to swallow—and I don't know that 'hemlock' maneuver."

"Heimlich," she corrects me, and then giggles.

Wow, a memory coup and an emotion, all wrapped up in one word. How can I get more of those? Just keep talking to her, I answer myself. At that moment, I'm gifted with an idea on how to proceed with Eve.

Meanwhile, dinner's over. "Let's wash the dishes before dessert. You clear, but don't carry any more than two things at a time." Naturally, she doesn't listen to me. But she does manage the task of transporting the dishes from the dining room to kitchen without incident.

"Now you go sit down at the table while I finish up washing. We're going to have story time before dessert."

Upon my return, I pop *Perry Como's Greatest Hits* into the CD player. He's so good for digestion, and I know Eve's been listening to him since she was a kid. Perry will help set the memory mood I want to create. Wish we had a fireplace. Outside the moon is lighting up our backyard with almost daytime brightness.

"Look at the cool moon shadows cast by the birches," I say, as I sit down. "And if you look beyond the icy harbor, you can even see moonbeams dancing on the waves. Sounds like a song title recorded by Perry, doesn't it, Eve? Cass will be calling soon, but first I'd like you to pay attention to what I say. We're going for a walk down memory lane. So look at me, please. This will only take about ten or 15 minutes, okay? Then you can chat with Cass and enjoy your ice cream reward, I mean, dessert.

"Eve, do you remember when we lived in Sedona, how much we enjoyed our getaways to Las Vegas, especially when Cass would fly in from Chicago to meet us? The first time we went it was springtime in Sedona, but still winter in Chicago. Cass needed a getaway. The fruit trees in our backyard were beginning to bud. We weren't so sure we wanted to leave at that time because everything was ready to blossom. The cacti were, too. Springtime in high desert country is such an awesome sight.

"Remember that huge pear cactus with its bright yellow flowers?" Eve nods enthusiastically. "And that the quail would lay their eggs right in the middle of it. We were sure it was to protect their babies from the coyotes. But I've never figured out how in the world they did it without stabbing themselves. Really weird, huh?"

Eve smiles and shakes her head. "Don't know."

"So, anyway, gambling fever must have bit us 'cause we did run off to Vegas. The temperature was in the sixties when we left, but a half-hour out of Sedona, and on our way to Flagstaff, it started to snow. In five minutes, we found ourselves in the middle of a blizzard. Remember? Cars were going off the road, accidents everywhere. Seemed like those crazy drivers thought snow was an invitation to speed. Scary, huh?"

Eve's eyes are open wide. Yep, she is remembering.

"But do we turn back? Heck no, we've got a date to meet Cass that night at the Barbary Coast. Glitzy it wasn't, but we loved that casino, didn't we? Remember we could actually open up our hotel room window? How novel. And all the Strip traffic noise and fumes came blowing in. Some fun, huh?"

Eve's staying with me, so I plow ahead.

"Anyway, this particular night we decided to stay at our casino. We were all pretty pooped from traveling. The Barbary Coast wasn't crowded and we had that whole bank of quarter double-bonus poker machines all to ourselves. Remember the three of us sitting along that wall?"

Do I detect a hint of gambling fever in Eve's eyes?

"So we're sitting there whooping it up. Probably sounded like we had a few too many. But there we were, chugging iced teas, taking turns rubbing each other's machines for luck. Cass had her own style. She'd caress that machine, coo at it, then slap it, and hit the button. She was the first to win the Aces jackpot.

"Well, with that, we all started, rubbing and slapping and coaxing and cooing at those machines. All of a sudden, one right after another, we got Aces. It was magic. Those machines kept spitting out jackpots all night."

Eve's rocking in her chair now, laughing along.

And then the phone rings. It's Cass. "Talk to Eve about Vegas," I urge her. "Sure, okay," comes the long-distance response. I put Eve on the phone, telling her who it is.

"Hi, Cass, we were just talking about the Barbary Coast," Eve says. And then she's giggling and snorting. "Oh, yeah, I remember that, too. Ha-ha. That's Donna for you."

It sounds to me like I'm the butt of some private joke. But who cares? Eve is actually animated.

Hallelujah! The conversation lasts almost five minutes. When Eve hangs up, I ask, "And who was that?"

She gives me a puzzled look like I'm the biggest dope in the world. "That was Cass. You know that, don't you?"

You betcha, Eve.

Eve retires to the living room with her chocolate almond ice cream to watch TV. I join her as a commercial comes on. Taking advantage of the minute, I nonchalantly ask her, "So what's new with Cass?"

"Huh, what?"

"Cass. You know the one you just talked to on the phone 15 minutes ago."

"Oh. I don't know. I forgot." Eve's eyes dart back to the TV screen. Well, that sure nipped that expectation in the bud.

"So what are you watching, Eve?"

"Um . . . I'm not sure. *Law and Order?*"

"Really? It's not Wednesday."

Eve looks at me quizzically.

"Never mind. I'll just sit with you." *Law and Order* it isn't. But that's okay. I really need the time to rethink what we may have accomplished tonight.

Maybe it's not the miracle of the century. But it is a start; the outcome was pretty good, and it's ideal to build on. I went fishing for an emotion and I caught several of them. If I keep doing it, I might land a big one. But, please, no expectations. Very dangerous to my mental health.

As the days progress, I hardly let a telephone call go by without doing my creative visualization/reminiscing routine. I even call a few friends and ask them to call Eve at an appointed time so I can do the exercise before the call. Then I tell Eve a story about her friend and sometimes show her a photo of one of their happy times together. I focus on the friend's unique personality characteristics and aim at getting an emotional reaction from Eve. I applaud Eve and reinforce any emotional responses by repeating what I overheard in her telephone conversation.

Perhaps more important, I repeat those victories to any of my friends who will listen. As important as it is to reinforce Eve's successes, in many ways it's more vital for me to reinforce mine. I need to know that I am accomplishing something. Anything.

Back in my beginning A.A. days, it was a tradition at my Friday night meeting to give out medallions commemorating anniversaries in sobriety. As I recall, one night when I was struggling to hang on to my one-year plus of sobriety, this guy announced he had ten years' sobriety. Seemed like a century to me. What an impossible dream. As was customary at that meeting, he delivered a minute-long speech on how he had accomplished his remarkable feat of ten continuous years of surrender to a Higher Power.

Here's the gist of what he said: "Many years ago, my sponsor told me that if I woke up with gratitude for a new day of sobriety, tried to keep that attitude alive during the day, then thanked God for my sobriety when I went to bed at night, I would never pick up a drink. The attitude of gratitude works."

His "advice" stunned me with its simplicity—and cunning. Of course, if a person is thinking "positive," a negative thought (or, in my case, the descent into self-pity or depression) hardly has a chance to take hold. This wasn't pop-psych-speak from some wishy-washy positive-thinking guru; this was a "from the trenches" strategy on how to stay sober one more day. Armed with the attitude of gratitude, I might not have to constantly go to war with those cravings and fearful thoughts that then seemed to dominate my days.

Later that night, I cozied up on my couch and wrote in my journal about the wise words I had heard. The more I wrote, the more I complicated his advice. But God was good to me. I knew from experience that a simple gratitude exercise might not capture my imagination long enough for it to become habitual. Here's the gratitude exercise I "invented": Every morning I would say (not necessarily believe) that I was grateful for the new day and looking forward to recounting later that night in my journal any moments of gratitude I would experience during the day.

Since I was mostly broke, irregularly working, didn't have family involvement or any love interest, I knew I had to dig pretty hard for reasons—other than my tentative sobriety—to be grateful to God for another day. So I decided to look for "miracles" in my daily life. Not big ones, just a little one or two.

For my gratitude-journaling purposes, I defined a miracle as anything "good" that happened to me that I did not directly cause. I decided to include happenings such as someone holding the door open as I exited the grocery store, or walking into the apartment building laundry room and discovering all the machines were immediately available, or (and this was a biggie) someone inviting me to coffee after an A.A. meeting and picking up the tab.

I figured if I could recount two or three of these "miracles" in my journal each day, I'd be doing pretty well. The first day, I was amazed. I recounted seven little miracles. For these, I was truly grateful. The next day, I had eight. This must be a fluke, I mused, as I happily recorded the events of the day. But it wasn't a fluke; the count never dipped below seven. Often it rose over ten, as I continued to record my simple life moments of gratitude over the next three or four years.

Why, oh why, did I stop that routine? My guess is that my life eventually got so good that it would've taken hours to record the little miracles of my day. But now, life is scary again. The thought of a drink has crossed my mind once too often in the past few months. It is time to resurrect the old attitude of gratitude routine . . . focusing on Eve's little successes as a brain-injury survivor and, more important, my triumphs as a rehabilitator/caregiver/homemaker and financial "wiz."

Perhaps inspired by my renewed interest in gratitude, I actually begin enjoying fishing for Eve's emotions. No matter how subtle Eve's response seems, I chalk it up as a victory. (Even a minnow can be used to catch a bigger fish.) The spark of recognition, the quick smile, and the nodding head all have become rewards in themselves for my efforts. Once I catch an emotion, I work it—repeating the line that inspired it, piling on more emotion or detail, asking Eve if she can remember what happened next—reinforcing the feeling in any way I can.

As long as I remain calm and positive, I can increase my awareness of Eve's behavior. All sorts of little rehabilitation triumphs are illuminated by that light. And they happen at the oddest moments. If I am overfocused on pursuing a rigid routine, or set my expectation level too high, I might miss them. The boring, deadly routine of it all will dull my senses—including the sixth, the one I am relying on more and more.

As we are taught in A.A., the "problem" is always me. So is the solution. By adjusting my perception of the rehabilitation problems as mine, I can begin looking for a solution, or new directions for my actions. I can't control Eve, the fallout from the brain aneurysm, or her rate of recovery. But all these elements are also part of my care-giving/rehabilitation problem. With permission to solve my problem, I have choices now: to respond or react to her behavior, or to continue on with whatever other right action is next on my agenda. This way I take the power out of a sick, unhealthy, situation and give it back to myself or, even better, turn it over to the care of a Higher Power.

As the days progress, Eve seems more alert, more often. When she tries to do something for herself, I most often let her. For instance, this morning she tried to blow-dry her own hair. Granted, this first attempt was a hairstyling disaster, but it gave her a choice and a decision to make. Does she want to look funny all day or re-wet her hair and try again? Since we are not going out, I can let go of that one and let her decide. She needs to begin again to experience life as a series of decisions or choices, all of which have consequences with which she will have to live. The same goes for those occasions when Eve resists my directions. Though I may be frustrated, I have to let her experience the consequences of her actions. And, since it's a "we" program, I benefit, too, as daily life delivers another growth "opportunity" to employ the program concept of letting go or—yippee!—practicing patience.

Despite the late-winter flurries, by mid-March there is more grass than snow showing on the Door County landscape. One morning, on our now daily march across the vacant lot to the post office, a brazen wildflower, boldly pushing up and out of the earth, catches my attention.

"Hey, look, Eve, an early spring surprise. Come and pick it. You can wear it in your buttonhole as a symbol of mutual survival. Gee, I wonder if the wildflowers are blooming along the Ridges nature trail. Of course, we can't pick those, but maybe I can take a picture or two. It'll be cool, especially if I can find some coming through the leftover snow. Like a treasure hunt. Yeah, let's go this afternoon."

The rest of the morning, I prep Eve for our field trip with books and pictures of wildflowers. It keeps her amused while I do the bills.

During lunch, I rehearse our trip, embellishing my monologue with whatever memories I can conjure up from past wildflower walks. I emphasize to Eve that the "grand prize" goes to whoever finds a wildflower in the snow so I can take my photo.

Soon enough, we're on site, strolling along the roadside trail. Ten or 15 minutes pass and I'm getting cold. So is Eve. I'm all set to call it a day when I catch sight of a perky purplish wildflower, popping out of the snow. Will Eve see it? Obviously, not without some help. Fortunately, subtlety is lost on her. I grab her shoulder and turn her around to face the treasure.

Eve points, with an emotion bordering on excitement. "I see one!" she exclaims.

"Good for you. Let me take a picture of you with your prize, and then we can go home for your reward. How about a nice steaming cup of hot chocolate 'cause, gosh darn, I'm freezing out here."

Back home, I recount our escapade while we warm up with hot chocolate. Then I plop her daily journal for speech therapy in front of her, with a direction to write a sentence or two about her find on the nature trail. "Put an emotion in those sentences."

"Dear Journal, Today I found a wildflower while walking with Donna. It felt good."

Poetry it ain't, but, at this stage, I'll take it.

As spring progresses, I surprise myself with how many interesting short field trips Door County offers. I can always count on some unusual nature find—be it flora or fauna. There's always something flying or hopping about to add enchantment to the experience. For my part, I do my best to dramatize the setting. Like an artist painting with words, I try to infuse it with over-the-top emotion. On our return home, I reinforce the moment by retelling the story, then having Eve record it in her journal. Still fishing for emotions, I try to help Eve keep everything we catch, somewhere in the depths of her subconscious.

A key element of my program is born of my advertising mentality. Whatever message I deliver to Eve, I am relentless about it. In other words, "I tell her what I'm going to say, then I tell her, then I tell her again what I said." Like a commercial for a bowl of cereal, I try to make mundane tasks come alive with all the snap, crackle, and pop I can muster.

Eve must be getting a little better, because one wintry spring day I discover that Eve has discovered fire: not the "rubbing two sticks together" orange variety, but rather the just-turn-a-knob, blue-flame kind. She said she wanted a cup of tea. I thought I was safe from having to teach her that yet because she did not grasp the microwave concept. Unfortunately, Eve found a teakettle and quickly figured out the first two-thirds of the water-heating process on the stove. It's the turning-off part she keeps forgetting.

I need to teach her a safety lesson fast. First, I decide to use a visualization approach in which one of our cats sets fire to its tail and burns down the house. The visualization ends up scaring me more than it scares Eve. So that doesn't work. Next I try catching Eve in the act, then scream and plead. But she still forgets. Before I follow through on my threat to remove the knobs, I try a combination approach. First, I print several "Beware of Danger" and "Remember to Turn Off the Stove" billboard-style posters, with a lovely picture of a burning cat tail. I post them on the wall over the stove. Each morning I warn her.

Then I enlist her sister-in-law to deliver the same warning over the phone, in case Eve is resisting a direct suggestion from me. I reinforce that with a daily suggestion: "Stay standing at the stove until the flame is turned off." As a last resort, any time she forgets the flame, I retrieve her tea and dump it down the sink. It takes a few weeks, but eventually it works.

One morning, while sipping coffee with Eve and watching the sunrise on the lake, I boldly decide we will tackle a new learning task. I ask Eve to pay attention. "Today we're going for a ride. We'll open the car windows and breathe in that almost summery air. Then we're going grocery shopping at Piggly Wiggly in Sister Bay.

"Yep, today's the day I believe I'll let you walk with me through the store. Exciting, huh? You can use the shopping cart to keep your balance. We will be buying bananas, milk, meat, veggies, and Rocky Road ice cream and cones. I'll show you where to find them. It'll be like a treasure hunt.

"Now, this trip is strategically planned to give you a bathroom break, if you need one. Luckily, there's a bathroom at the 'Pig.' The trick is to tell me if you need to go. Do you think you can pay attention to that feeling? We're going to try and stay dry today, right? So tell me if you feel an urge."

"I will, I promise," Eve says determinedly.

Most people never give grocery shopping a second thought. But, speaking as one prone to anxiety attacks, I can vouch for the pop-psych fact that a routine trip to the grocery store can be an overwhelming, anxiety-producing experience. No other ordinary environment is purposely designed to be so confusing and overstimulating to the senses. Many an anxiety-attack sufferer tells the tale of abandoning a half-filled shopping cart and racing out of the store, gulping fresh air as she races for the safety of her car. For many years, I would not even attempt grocery shopping without first fortifying myself with liquid courage. I know I am not the only one who regularly shopped in an alcoholic stupor.

But back to my rehab challenge. Eve will eventually need to go grocery shopping. I can make this as serene as possible by drawing on my own experience in relearning to shop sober, plus my knowledge of how supermarkets are designed to encourage impulse buying.

I tell Eve, "In preparation for our first shopping trip, we're going to make a list. We'll construct it to match the store's layout. We'll use the weekly shopping guide from the newspaper to see what's on sale, but we won't let in-store sales sway our decisions. If it's not on the list, we won't buy it.

"We won't dilly-dally as we walk through. On this trip, I'll show you exactly where our staple items are located. Meanwhile, you keep your eyes focused on the aisles. Try to concentrate on following our route, rather than looking at all the items on the shelves. We'll be making a beeline from one item on our list to the next. I've included several treats on our list that we can afford to buy. That's enough for this shopping trip. Agreed? Okay, let's get ready."

Along the route to the Piggly Wiggly, I notice that Door County is springing up all over. Nowadays I never pass up an opportunity to embellish the obvious with a creative play-by-play commentary.

"Look at the cobalt blue sky, Eve, and all the cotton-ball clouds gathering in the west. Uh-oh. Do you think a storm's brewing? Hear that? I think it was frog croaks. Of course, we just went over the creek. Look up there. Is it a hawk, maybe an eagle? Tell me what you think." And so on.

When we arrive at the "Pig," I hand the list to Eve. "You're in charge of checking it off. But before we go in, let's take three deep breaths and relax. It's a big moment for you. Let's go."

# 17

# Follow the Bouncing Ball

Easter Sunday brunch at a fancy Door County restaurant. At face value, Jennifer and her husband's invitation is a kind, loving, Christian gesture. But a little voice in my head sabotages that feeling by proclaiming, "Hey, it's a test!"

Will Eve overstuff her mouth with food, forcing me to make her spit it out? Will she cut her food into small, manageable pieces, or choke on a chunk of ham? Will she be incontinent, flatulent, burp, belch, or snort? Will she yawn incessantly, or just grin and look stupid, or actually try to participate in conversation? Will I just burst into tears in memory of all the happier Easters past, where going out to dinner was a treat and not a test of my rehabilitation prowess?

It's our first invitation out with friends. If I dwell on the possibilities in Eve for socially unacceptable behavior, I will talk myself out of going. So, okay, maybe she's not ready. But then maybe this opportunity to rise to a social occasion is just the sort of spark Eve's psyche needs to propel her to a new level of social awareness. For sure, it could provide a new emotional connection to past holiday celebrations for us to work on.

What to do? I call Eve into the dining room. "Please pay attention, Eve. I have some exciting news. This will only take a minute." I pause to let some anticipation build. "Guess what? Jennifer and Jim want us to join them for Easter Sunday brunch at Alexander's. It's a very chi-chi restaurant in Sister Bay. Would you like to go?"

Eve nods enthusiastically. This is good.

"Okay. But you understand we'll have to dress up and look pretty. Perhaps we'll rouge your lips with a little lipstick, eh? And you'll have to mind your table manners. I won't be able to constantly tell you to chew three times, swallow, and then sip some water. They'll get very bored and it will be embarrassing to do that. Will you watch how you eat, all by yourself? If you accidentally burp or make any body noises, you'll say 'excuse me,' won't you? It's only polite. We don't want to disrupt their holiday dinner, do we? For one thing, it's expensive. We're going to elevate our behavior. Gosh, I hope I can remember not to belch or snort in public. 'Errp, snoort, aagh.'"

Eve giggles at my boorish interjection.

"Okay. We'll try not to do that. Agreed? Now I'll call Jennifer back and we'll accept their invitation."

Except for a flat tire, our Easter outing is a success. Thank God for those patient people who put up with Eve's halting conversations and my anxious watchfulness on our first social ventures.

The final Friday in April, Graduation Day at NEW presents me with a mixed bag of emotions. On the one hand, I'm happy that the three-times-a-week trek to Green Bay is over. On the other hand, Eve hasn't progressed that much in my book; she's still barely capable of coping with everyday life.

I invite Cass to Door County to commemorate the occasion. NEW's occupational therapist, Pattie, has helped Eve plan and prepare a celebration lunch. The three of us are gathered in the occupational therapy kitchen, watching Eve slowly assemble salami sandwiches. She adds a final touch of pickle garnish and successfully serves her feast. It's a melancholy moment for me. Sure, it beats spoon-feeding her; but if this is as good as it gets, I'm not sure I can handle it.

After lunch we all attend Eve's final staffing. The always-positive Pattie makes a big deal out of Eve's lunch-making success as well as her amazing vacuuming skills. The physical therapists are pleased with Eve's increased stamina, the loosening of her "frozen" shoulder, and her slightly improved balance. The speech therapist, however, speaks of her frustration. She had discontinued Eve's therapy session several weeks prior because of Eve's resistance to recording events in a daily journal. The therapist notes that Eve is highly capable of comprehending what she reads and is also able to quickly solve logic problems (a lot quicker than I, in most instances). The therapist predicts, though, that Eve's resistance to journaling will certainly hinder the return of her short-term memory function. She predicts Eve will continue to confuse short- and long-term memories, a condition Eve self-corrects by confabulating.

Next the psychological counselor notes Eve's continual lack of emotional response. On the plus side, Eve doesn't appear to be depressed. The counselor also voices her concern over our relatively isolated living situation in Baileys Harbor and the possibility of caregiver burnout. She makes me promise to make arrangements for a "sitter" so that I can attend A.A. meetings more frequently.

The rehabilitation physician recites the litany of medications for controlling a variety of Eve's problems including her inability to focus, depression, the high blood pressure condition acquired post aneurysm, and the possibility of more seizures. He'll check Eve's progress in a month or so.

Lastly, the admissions director speaks, noting that no further rehabilitation is required at this time. I mentally note that this is fortunate, because—"coincidentally"—Eve has used up all of her rehabilitation insurance coverage for the year.

And then the staffing meeting is over. We're free. Cass and Eve take off down the hall as I lag behind to walk with the admissions director. I will miss her calming influence on me. She has been helpful and concerned above and beyond the call of duty since day one. While we walk, both of us are watching Eve zigzag down the hall, bouncing off Cass and, occasionally, the wall. When we reach the door, the director pats my arm, wishes me good luck, and invites me to call her if the need arises. Then she adds, "I'm afraid Eve has come as far as she's going to."

My stomach lurches. I manage to smile and proffer the appropriate "Thank you, and goodbye." But once outside the facility, my temper flares. For my mental health, I know I can't afford to believe that. "You are so wrong," I defiantly announce to the bright spring day that awaits us. Cass and Eve pay no attention to my mutterings. I guess I talk to myself a lot these days.

Cass stays on through the unexpectedly gorgeous weekend. Nature's celebration of the last days of winter and valiant effort to come alive again in spring is one of Door County's best-kept secrets. Of course, the tourist brochures proclaim the wondrous display of cherry and apple blossoms across the peninsula. But my favorite spring sightings are the myriad wildflowers that dot the peninsula. They are everywhere and anywhere, nature's tiniest treasures hidden in unmowed lawns, pushing through cracks in sidewalks, and peeking out from underneath rusty wheelbarrows. Or, if I need a quick fix, I can find oodles of them dancing on the forest floors or boldly punctuating green pastures. I've even come to view lowly dandelions in a new light, especially the sight of thousands of yellow sunbursts carpeting a farmer's field. Quite a show each spring—and best of all, it's free.

After Cass heads back for Chicago, Eve and I resume our daily non-routine. Try as I might, I just can't discipline myself to organize the day by the clock. Consequently, I pay by regularly overthinking my daily plan of action for executing the mostly dull duties. Life would be easier if I weren't so rebellious. Ah, I guess the best I can do is accept who I am . . . and keep asking my Higher Power and subconscious for help.

As May rolls over into June, our patio doors are once again open to the lake breeze and the ever-soothing sounds of lapping waves and calling seagulls. With the promise of summer, Eve's eyes seem more sparkly, her mind more alert, her speech a bit more animated. In addition to our daily jaunt to the post office, we're going for longer walks in and out of town. Baileys Harbor is already bustling with tourists.

Life would be so deadly dull without this change of seasons. We have two in Door County: winter and springsummerfall, aka tourist season. I've tried to expand my mind and believe that Wisconsin has four separate seasons, but honestly, there seems to be only a four-week stretch on either end of summer when we are confidently snow-free. Sorry, tourist bureau, but snow equals winter . . . and one month of snowlessness does not a season make.

As usual, May combines the best—and worst—of Marchaprilmay. Finally, the daffodils are in bloom, but then, so are the lilacs. Today everyone is celebrating Memorial Day, perhaps in memory of the warmth of sunshine. Those who managed to dodge raindrops and to plant all of their spring flowers last weekend get to enjoy the big tourist season kickoff: Maifest in Jacksonport.

Jacksonport likes to call itself "the quiet side." Usually it is. I'm quite fond of the town. It reminds me of the way most of Door County was 40 years ago: a few stores, a couple of bars, and classy restaurants off the main drag. In the center of town is a big grassy park with a path that heads down to a sandy beach on the lake. A cool breeze rustles the new leaves of the huge old shade trees while the sun warms us up in between the morning shadows.

The town sponsors an art fair of sorts. Actually, most of the peninsula artists have their own galleries that they're tending to, but if you look around, you can find some local color interspersed with the professional traveling crafter booths at the Jacksonport show.

This will be Eve's post-aneurysm debut on the Door County festival scene. It should be relatively safe; the only danger I'm concerned about is her losing her balance next to a ceramics display.

It's a 15-minute drive from Baileys Harbor, which for me is the highlight of the outing. Thanks to last night's rain, the spring colors are sparkling in the morning sun. I try to make a mental note of all the different "greens" I see, but it's nigh impossible. What a soothing solution for bathing winter-weary eyes! Has the sky ever been bluer? Though there's a gathering of gray-purple rain clouds on the southwest horizon, the creamy clouds above us are blushing. A barely perceptible rosy light makes them appear incandescent.

Almost there. Tourists' cars are parked along the side of the road. Even though we're a half-mile out, we'd better look for a parking place now. We end up parking next to a forested area. The cacophonic calls of blue jays greet us as we disembark. I guess the jays are not used to tourists in this locale, and they're protesting our invasion. We join the tourist parade to the Jacksonport Park. The scent of cedars intermingles with the aroma of carnival confections as we draw closer.

I say to Eve, "The schedule of events says there's a fish boil at noon. Would you like an early dinner today, or would you rather save up the experience for our favorite fish boil restaurant, maybe next weekend?"

Eve stops to ponder, as if thinking, talking, and walking would be too much for her brain. "Next week," she eventually answers.

Hmm. A wise decision and an extraordinary act of delayed gratification. It's hard to pass up a fish boil, Door County's famous culinary delight. Just imagining it makes my mouth water. The traditional fish boil is an outdoor happening that I never tire of watching.

The Boilmaster begins by building a roaring fire, using wood. As he stokes the fire, he gives this spiel to the crowd of hungry spectators: "In the bubbling cauldron before you, we're boiling little red potatoes and onions. They've been cooking about 15 minutes now, so it's almost time to add the fresh whitefish."

On cue, his two assistants enter, toting a mesh basket filled with more than enough whitefish to feed the crowd. As they lower it into the cauldron, the Boilmaster explains that the three ingredients will cook for another ten minutes.

Now, some serious stoking begins. The crowd backs up as the fire blazes. And then it's time to get ready for the climax. "Okay, folks. Now comes everyone's favorite part: the boilover. You boys keep the

171

fire going good. You folks back up a little, 'cause I'm throwing kerosene on the fire. The pot will boil over, taking the fish oils with it. Ready? One, two, three." WHOOSH! The fire flares. Flames leap skyward. The spectators ooh and ahh as they retreat. And the assistants race to take out the fish and vegetables.

The next thing you know, you're looking down at an incredible feast: melt-in-your-mouth fish, robust potatoes, and sublime onions, all swimming in melted butter. Nothing compares to this succulent blend of flavors, especially when they're accompanied by homemade rye bread, coleslaw, and a frosty beer. (Oops, did I say that? I meant iced tea.)

As if things couldn't get any better, dessert is always homemade cherry pie topped with vanilla ice cream. Drool.

"Hey, Eve, are you sure you don't want the fish boil?" Oh, don't say that, Donna. You'll sway her. "Never mind, Eve. But I think we better have some breakfast. See that booth over there? The sign says cherry pie à la mode, $2.50. Let's go for it. We can go sit at a picnic table on the beach and pig out."

"Yeah," Eve says, with one of her biggest bursts of emotion all week. "Sounds good to me."

"What a beautiful day," I exclaim, in between cherry pie bites. "Just look at all the variations of blue in that lake: silvery cerulean by the shore rocks, then turquoise, Prussian blue where it gets deep, and then, oh I don't know, Prussian green, maybe. Hmm, I don't think there is such a color, Eve. Don't bother remembering that."

She isn't paying any attention to me anyway. She's busy people-watching, something that holds minimal fascination for me versus nature-watching. I make a mental note that I should take her out more often to do her thing. "All done, Eve? Let's go back and see the rest of the craft show."

It's another lazy summer morning, and I'm stuck inside, doing laundry and paying portions of bills. Eve hasn't budged from the dining room table. She's been staring out the dining room window for an hour now. I suggest she think about getting dressed for a walk to the post office. She looks at me with glazed eyes and robotically nods.

What's the matter with her, I wonder. She seems so unresponsive. And she's been acting dopier for several days now. She yawns all the time. Maybe her brain shunt is clogged? Maybe she needs more Ritalin?

Well, I sure as heck don't know those answers. I'd better bite the bullet and call her rehab physician in Green Bay. I dread the calling process. I always feel like a hysterical woman, overreacting to normal broken-brain behavior. If I only knew what to expect. To make matters worse, I never get the doctor on the first try and the receptionist never seems to get my message correct. I feel like giving up before I start.

But today is miraculously different. Not only is the doctor "in," he'll even speak to me if I hang on for a minute. Whoa, the stars are smiling on me.

"Hi, doctor. I might have a problem with Eve. I'm not sure. She seems dopier the past few days. Do you know what I mean? That's right, not as responsive. Lethargic? Oh yeah. So I was wondering, do you think maybe she needs to have the Ritalin increased, or maybe the shunt is blocked?

"You don't think it's the shunt? Wait, you'd better repeat that for me because I don't understand. You're saying that too much Ritalin can cause her to act dopey like this? You think she might not need it anymore and now it's working in reverse? Okay, so now what? Wean her off the Ritalin. Okay, we'll try that first. Yes, I'll watch her closely."

I hang up the phone, shaking my head in disbelief. Wouldn't you think someone would have warned me about the consequences of too much Ritalin? I wasn't told to watch out for this. I didn't even know you could "overdose" by taking it as prescribed. For crying out loud, this is a heavy-duty drug, a controlled substance. Thank goodness I called. Even though I still have to deal with Eve's dopiness, my mood quickly switches from free-floating anxiety to buoyant hopefulness. To celebrate, I allow myself the pleasure of thinking— something I've tried hard to avoid.

I ponder the possibilities of a life without Ritalin. I don't dare go online at this point and overwhelm myself with too much information. Instead, I work with what I know. Remembering my objections and confusion when it was initially prescribed for Eve, I review what the doctors told me. Contrary to my original belief, Ritalin doesn't act like a sedative to calm down kids with attention-deficit problems; instead, it's supposed to help stimulate their brains, thereby decreasing their need for hyperactivity to amuse themselves. It's a stimulant. If Eve no longer needs it, then the outside world must be getting through to her brain.

I go one step further with my thoughts. When Dr. Larry Beuret switched the focus of his medical practice from psychosomatic disorders to attention disorders, the first case histories he gave me to help in my writing his patient information brochures almost never mentioned hyperactivity as a primary symptom. If anything, the patients were depressed, lethargic, and often suffering from anxiety attacks.

In preparation for switching his practice, Dr. Beuret had traveled to England to study with a group of doctors who were using precision eye exercises to alleviate the symptoms and help correct the problems of attention disorders. Dr. Beuret gave me their studies for background; I only partially understood them.

In fact, since I was in early sobriety at the time, the portions of the studies that fascinated me most were the discussions of anxiety symptoms and the correction of tunnel vision. Like many alcoholics, I desperately wanted a medical or psychological cure for my ailment. Anything was preferable to simply quitting drinking.

I vaguely remembered an alcoholism study from some revered East Coast university or medical college. It said that the one physical symptom all alcoholics shared across the board was a significantly above-average tendency toward tunnel vision in their testing situations. I could certainly relate to that finding. Heck, if I didn't keep my eyes constantly moving while driving over a bridge or on one of those out-in-space cloverleaf expressway exits, I wouldn't be here to talk about it.

I came away from my background reading with a fuzzy understanding that anxiety, inner-ear imbalance, and tunnel vision were all somehow connected with the inability to focus attention correctly.

Back to the present. I can't be certain if Eve has an anxie[ty prob]lem because the antidepressant and the seizure-control medicine probably effectively masking it. But for certain, she does have a balance problem, and she always looks like she's doing that tunnel-vision thing. And to complicate matters, her ongoing struggle with that frozen shoulder has affected her ability to turn her head easily. Not that she can't, if I point it out. It's more like something inside her tells her that it is safer not to do it.

Though I make all these intellectual connections, I fail to make the leap by calling Dr. Beuret for his opinion. Instead, I decide to wait for my scheduled follow-up call to the rehabilitation doctor in three days. I make a note to myself to ask if he is aware of a connection between balance problems, attention disorders, and eye exercises.

Three days later, I can hardly believe I'm excited about calling the doctor. When we finally connect, I dump all my theories and conclusions on him in one breathless thousand-word sentence.

I'm floored when he says he knows what I'm talking about. In fact, he says, "There's a physical therapist in Green Bay who runs a balance and dizziness clinic." He believes she uses hand-eye coordination exercises as part of her rehabilitation routine. If I'd like, he'll prescribe a couple of sessions for Eve.

Well, duh, yeah. Geez, how come I had to ask instead of being told? It's a constant thought I long ago decided wasn't worth repeating to anyone involved in the conventional healthcare industry.

The next day we're on the road to the balance and dizziness clinic in Green Bay. I'm so happy I'm not even worried about lack of insurance coverage. Just give me those eye exercises!

When we arrive, Eve's balance is tested with some ordinary physical therapy and a fancy, big-bucks apparatus that spits out a string of statistics that verifies her balance is way off. But as the therapist explains, there's really no absolute way to know whether the problem lies in Eve's visual perception, or in the brain's processing of her visual perception, or in the communications the brain delivers back that allow her body to adapt to the environmental cues. I interpret this finding as "no way you two can afford to get that answer."

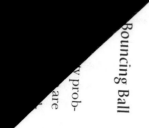

owever. I'm going for symptom correction, not about the eye exercises?" I ask.

we recommend," she responds, as she hands copied pages of oh-so-simple hand-eye coordi- continues, "Have her do these faithfully twice a day for six weeks and see if there's any improvement. If not, come back and we'll try something else."

We do not go back, mainly because the improvement from the simple exercises is, quite frankly, astounding. When I say simple, I mean easy and fast—15 minutes max. Most are variations on the "follow the bouncing ball" theme. Just watching Eve do the exercises propels me into a zone. I'm on a high of hope, inspired by the uncharacteristic feeling of confidence that fills me. For the first time in this whole ordeal, I believe that I'm finally doing something in terms of rehab that is actually going to work.

As those early summer days progress, so does Eve. Whether it's the Ritalin detoxification or the eye-exercise addition, I'm not sure. But she seems more alert, better able to focus, and she's yawning less throughout the day.

We begin a new era in rehabilitation one fine Saturday morning. Breakfast is over. I'm about to toss a load of dirty clothes into the washer when a great new idea dawns in my little brain.

"Eve, today I'm going to teach you how you used to do the laundry." I rub my hands with fiendish glee. I hate doing laundry; once upon a time it was Eve's favorite household chore. The only trick will be my remembering her persnickety way of sorting, double rinsing, and employing several different cleaning aids. My way is to stuff as much into the washer as possible. Her way elevates the term "housework" to the status of domestic engineering.

I rifle through the desk and find my teaching tools: 3x5 index cards and several different colored pens.

"Here, Eve, you'll take notes while I dictate to you how I believe you used to do the laundry. But first let's take three deep breaths and relax." (I'm going to require a lot of subconscious help remembering Eve's routine.) "Now I want you to interrupt me, Eve, if any direction I give you sounds contrary to your old way of doing things. Ready? Let's start with the basic hot whites."

I've written a slew of "how-to" instructions in the course of my advertising career, so I don't know why I am surprised that three hours later I am still dictating the dozens of individual steps involved in the sorting/washing/drying process. Finally, I announce to Eve, "It's a wrap. And, God, I need a nap. How about you? We'll execute the laundry task tomorrow. I've had it for today."

Initially, I hover over Eve's shoulder every step of the way on laundry day. Gradually, I let go of controlling, trusting she'll use the cue cards as a guide. Sometime during the next few weeks, I hear a washing machine going while I find myself staring at the cue cards, nearly buried under a pile of bills. Lord knows how many loads Eve has done without the cue cards to guide her! I'm all set to scream when I realize that I'm wearing clean clothes. So what's the problem, Donna? If it's not broke, don't fix it. Duh.

# 18

# Typical One-Day Plan

I myself never routinely followed a written plan because I wasn't consciously aware that I had developed a strategy for either brain rehabilitation or caregiver coping. As you have seen, for the most part, I interacted with Eve on an intuitive (subconscious) level that first year. Written routines and conscious planning did not become part of our daily lives until two years into her recovery.

The following one-day plan, developed circa eight months into Eve's recovery, is brought to you in hindsight.

To begin, I did—still do—make a conscious commitment to live one day at a time. Actually, I try to compartmentalize the day into morning, afternoon, and evening segments. This conscious action helps me hold my expectations in check.

Over breakfast, I would listen to Eve read aloud from three spiritual daily meditation books. At least one of these focused on 12-Step program concepts. After Eve wrote a one-sentence summary of each meditation in her daily journal, I'd ask her for comments. We would discuss the day's lessons for about ten minutes. If I didn't hear something to help me motivate Eve, I'd hear the words I needed for myself. There are no such things as coincidences, are there?

Afterward, I'd retreat to the backyard bluff overlooking the lake. (Actually, any quiet place would do.) I'd take three deep breaths to quiet my mind, followed by a prayer announcing my willingness to align my will with the Almighty's. I'd admit (and try to accept) my powerlessness over the caregiving situation. I'd invite my Higher Power to walk with me through the day's routine and help me through any surprises life might present. Then I'd decide on my next right action(s) for the coming hours, reminding myself not to entertain any expectations for the outcomes of my actions.

All of these calming exercises worked to take my conscious analytical mind out of the picture and give my subconscious free rein. Afterward, I'd contemplate the lake for a while waiting for an answer or direction from the heavens—perhaps an intuitive thought, maybe an "ah-ha" realization, or, if nothing else, a feeling that I could go back inside and continue through the day with some semblance of sanity. Then throughout the day, I'd continue "conversing" with my Higher Power, asking for help or checking my motives and my never-ending tendency to try to control situations.

After meditation, I'd look in on Eve, who was usually at some early stage of dressing herself in preparation for her daily walk to the post office. If I felt confident enough in her ability to react to environmental cues that day, I'd let her walk to the post office alone to retrieve our mail from the P.O. box. Generally speaking, I encouraged self-sufficiency, even if it made me nervous. I had to work at letting go of my worries, especially when her safety—or mine—was at stake.

About this time in Eve's recovery, a neighbor reported that she had seen Eve cross the state highway without looking both ways. I was grateful for the feedback. I sensed that other people's negative opinions about her ability to cross the street had more impact on Eve's subconscious than the obvious personal safety issue, so I used it on her.

As usual, anytime Eve "relapsed" to incorrect behavior, I took her back to the previous rehab stage. I also explained to her why I was doing this. As Eve and I walked to the curb to rehearse the "look both ways" routine, I said, "From now on, everyone in town will be watching you cross the street . . . and you can bet I'm paying them to tattle on you. Don't embarrass yourself by not paying attention while crossing a busy street. Do you want to embarrass me by making me look like a neglectful caregiver? . . . I didn't think so. So here's the plan. Whenever you reach the curb, I want you to exaggerate the action of looking both ways . . . like this. Then all the busybodies in town can clearly see that you know how to cross a street."

Eventually, it became a habit. Incidentally, I noted that the idea of exaggerating the action also helped to impress Eve's subconscious with its importance. In fact, stopping any routine action in the middle of it, then exaggerating it by making a joke or overdramatizing it, is always helpful for impressing the subconscious with its importance. It's a handy teaching tool in a variety of rehabilitation situations.

After her walk, Eve would take a tea break and I would give her a project, centered in one room. For example, cleaning the living room always required vacuuming, dusting, and cleaning tabletops. We practiced the steps involved in every project side by side for a week or two. When she was able to complete the project successfully alone, she was allowed, or more often directed, to do it on her own. (Actually, I usually ended up having to "motivate" her every 15 minutes or so.)

Practicing projects together is simply the "act as if" concept in action. Because our "actions" were intertwined, it became a setup for success. I happily gave Eve all the credit for a job well done.

At some point in the middle of teaching a project, we would have sessions where I would dictate every how-to step of a project as Eve took notes on index cards or in a notebook. As a way of reviewing, Eve would "talk" the steps back to me. That way, I could see which areas were unclear in her mind. We did these step-by-step verbal project reviews several times during the project-teaching process. This is simply a variation on that age-old advertising technique: "Tell them what you're going to say, then tell them, then tell them again to remind them what you just told them."

Every time I assigned a project or task, I would link it with a secondary gain, that is, the satisfaction of a need or reinforcement of a value Eve held dear. For example, the suggestion to shower (which Eve resisted in the early days) would be coupled with, "You want to look nice if we run into somebody at the store," or (more crudely) "You don't want to stink up our A.A. meeting." As time went on, my suggestion would be phrased as, "You should take a shower, Eve. Why? Because . . ." Then I'd pause and allow her to fill in the blanks aloud. Subconsciously speaking, this was most impressive.

Conversely, I also tried to align any "corrections of mistakes" in terms of her value system. For example, if Eve did a sloppy job of dusting the living room, I'd ask her how she'd feel if friends popped in unexpectedly and saw that smeared coffee-table top. Knowing Eve, I believed that inviting guests into a clean house, a point of pride all her life, was far more important than other motivations such as "Dirt is a health hazard," or "Cleanliness is next to godliness," or "Here's a good occupational therapy exercise for you, Eve."

Continuing through our typical day, Eve would take a one- to two-hour nap after lunch. Since she was never a napper in the "old days," I'd reinforce that suggestion with, "It's time to recharge your brain batteries, or else you'll be dopey by dinnertime. If that happens, then I'll be forced to fix it instead of you. How do peanut butter and jelly sandwiches sound?" It was such a heartless, empty threat that I could barely keep from smiling. Judging from Eve's smirk, I knew I couldn't fool her either. This brings me to another point.

Early on, I discovered that Eve did have remnants of her old sense of humor. For that, I was very grateful. I played to it all the time. Nothing disarms the resistant mind faster than a chuckle. Humor is also a great vehicle for teaching a lesson or motivating behavior change. Just look at all the funny TV commercials. Believe me, the advertiser is well aware of the power of humor. Otherwise, he wouldn't be spending big bucks to camouflage his dead-serious message to buy his product in the fluff and puff of a humorous approach.

Back to the all-important nap. If, for some reason, I couldn't convince Eve to sleep, I still enforced a rest period by playing one of those environmental nature sounds tapes while she "closed her eyes" for an hour. Then I'd lie down next to her and promptly fall asleep, proving beyond doubt that something worked.

Upon waking, Eve would be given another task, usually a continuation of the morning project or a task she already knew how to do. I limited teaching new tasks to one a day.

That would bring us up to "fun time" at four o'clock, an hour dedicated to exercising Eve's brain. Generally, we worked a crossword puzzle together, not that I was ever much help. (I'm pretty sure my subconscious resisted the idea of supplying someone else's idea of the "right" word.) But whenever Eve got stuck on a word, I would attempt to give her alternate clues. Even if I was guessing wrong, it was still a brain exercise for Eve to match a word with my clue or definition. At five, we would check the solutions at the back of the book. Eve was instructed to look in the dictionary for any words that I deemed should be part of her vocabulary and record their definitions in a journal. (In my opinion, Scrabble would have served our purposes better, but, unfortunately, it didn't work with just two of us.)

Afterward, our attention turned to "What's for dinner?" and the prerequisite task of meal preparation. Suffice it to say that Eve stood by my side in the kitchen and watched me prepare dinner until the experience was just too agonizing for her. As I've pointed out, the subconscious mind is most concerned with survival, so Eve's subconscious was highly motivated to take over dinner prep as soon as it was able.

After dinner and dessert, we would set off on a "fishing for emotions" expedition into the subconscious. This exercise involved a mixture of stories from our past and creative visualizations, all designed to evoke an emotional response from Eve.

The storytelling part centered on an incident involving an old friend, a vacation episode, or some joyous, memorable social occasion. The creative visualization aspect was my attempt to arouse Eve's sensory memories, which are generally strongly linked to emotions in the subconscious mind. For example, in describing an event from our Cancún vacation, a dinner on the patio of a seaside restaurant, I tried to recall aspects of the event that were obviously perceived by one of the five senses. As always, I infused my story with "over the top" emotion.

"Remember, it was a warm night in January . . . ha-ha," I began. "Can you believe we were actually grateful to be cooled by the Caribbean breeze? Come on, we'll pretend we're there. Let's breathe in that salty sea air. Ready? Ah . . . Now let's watch the waves as they lap at the shore. Any moment now, the moon will pop out of the water. Let's hope it's a big round one.

"Yessirree. Remember, there was that strolling mariachi band. I think they played 'Coo Coo Paloma' for us." I sing a few bars as Eve winces. "Oh, now this was embarrassing. Remember, we didn't have money to tip them 'cause we were packing plastic that night. Then there was that coconut drink the waiter wanted us to try? You thought it would be too sweet, but it had a surprising twist. It was tangy. Come on, admit it, Eve. It was yummy, wasn't it? I think we ordered sea bass that night. Actually, I believe I had sea bass every night. Delicious. They fixed it a thousand different ways. It melted in your mouth, remember?"

Details, details. I surprised myself by how many details my subconscious came up with for these visualizations. But I was extremely motivated to see any kind of light in Eve's eyes. Thankfully, my subconscious responded with the sensory memories I needed to trigger an emotional response from Eve.

Cass always telephoned after dessert. I would usually prompt Eve to ask Cass a question or relate an incident from earlier in the day. Then, of course, she and Cass would discuss it on the phone. Afterward, I would ask Eve for Cass's comments. I never really got much of a response, nor was I able to convince her to take notes during phone conversations.

After many frustrating attempts, I gave up. Much later, I attributed this behavior to Eve's years of experience as an A.A. sponsor, where conversations are considered confidential. As a rule, I never quizzed her about the content of phone calls, especially with sponsees such as Cass. Obviously, Eve's subconscious still thought her phone calls were none of my business.

That was okay. My rehabilitation goal was not to create a "new" Eve, but to bring back "old" Eve behaviors by aligning my subconscious suggestions with her lifelong beliefs, needs, and values. I had more than enough avenues to explore with that.

Ethically speaking, I would be out of line if my motivation were to change old habits, including the ones that annoyed me, without Eve's stated desire and/or expressed willingness to change. She was not capable of offering either at this stage. Not to worry, though. As the supreme protector of the self, Eve's subconscious had no problem telling me to stay away from its sacred territory, by stubbornly resisting my attempts to change any behavior it considered essential for Eve's emotional/spiritual survival.

As the evening progressed, Eve would finally be free to indulge in her favorite "bad habits," most of which were at odds with everything I hoped to accomplish during the day for brain rehabilitation. At eight months, Eve had resumed her old habit of watching TV while reading a newspaper and/or a book or two. (On the positive side, every *Law and Order* rerun from that period seemed like a fresh, new episode to her.) Generally speaking, multitasking with brain damage does not help one develop good habits for improving memory.

All things considered, I believed it was more important for Eve to enjoy her "free time" without enduring a nightly inquisition from the rehabilitator. I did limit the amount of time she spent on the computer to a half-hour, however. Any more than that and Eve would zone out. Solitaire and "surfing the net" were Eve's addictions before the aneurysm. Frankly, I didn't have the energy to battle an addiction in addition to brain damage. So if logic or pleading didn't work, I simply shut down the computer when her time was up.

By ten o'clock, Eve would be ready for bed.

On the other hand, I would stay up and enjoy the carefree hours until midnight. Though I rarely surfed the Internet anymore for rehabilitation ideas, I did search for puzzles and memory books that might intrigue Eve . . . then on to the computer card games. Before retiring, I would jot down the day's successes, surprises, and little miracles in my gratitude journal. Then the cats and I would trot off to bed. I'd say a little prayer for continued sobriety, sanity, and serenity (of sorts), then ask my subconscious to help me solve this or that problem while I slept. Not one of my bedtime petitions ever went unanswered.

# 19

# A Dream Come True

My second-favorite holiday is fast approaching. The Baileys Harbor Fourth of July celebration rivals the corniest Hollywood recreation of America's birthday.

The big day dawns as beautiful as any summer day ever glorified in a poem. A rosy red sun is showering dazzling white sparkles on the deepest blue lake, and everything is waving in the breeze, just like Old Glory. In fact, the whole town is pulsating with excitement because at 9 A.M. the annual parade begins. Macy's it ain't. But small-town America still puts on the best show—with a high school marching band, red-faced politicians throwing candy out of convertibles, kids being pulled by costumed dogs, and a local plumber towing a banner-festooned outhouse.

Eve and I head down to the bottom of our long driveway, lawn chairs in hand. Even though we're half an hour early, we have to fight for good positioning on our own property. That's the way it goes. It's an accepted fact that all lakefront property is public domain for viewing the Fourth of July festivities.

I remind Eve that she is not a child, so please don't scramble with the kids to grab a piece of free-flying candy. Much to my chagrin, I find myself breaking my own rule an hour later as I dive for a fireball jawbreaker rolling my way on the pavement. Everybody—even sophisticated Chicago tourists—gets in the spirit for the parade, applauding the town's five aging members of the VFW and cheering on the volunteer firemen atop a shiny new fire truck. It's our town's pride and joy, don't you know?

The night before, Cass had called with a spur-of-the-moment announcement that she was driving up. She planned to leave Chicago at 5 A.M. so she could participate in Eve's first lucid holiday since the aneurysm. But now the parade's almost over and Cass is nowhere in sight. I'm worried, but there's nothing I can do at the moment. There's a parade blocking our driveway.

Finally, the last homemade float chugs past our personal reviewing stand. The crowd stands up in unison, dusts off its collective behind, and folds up the temporary seating.

I hurry Eve back to the house, hoping Cass has called on her cell phone and left us a message as to why she's delayed. Yep, the answering machine is blinking. I punch the button and am greeted by a string of cuss words sputtered in Cass's familiar drawl. "I should have been there at 8:30, but the county police blocked off every damned road that leads to Baileys Harbor. I know. I've been up and down those county trails for an hour, trying to find a way into town. Now I'm parked at that blue-collar bar on 57. I'm not alone, but everybody in the parking lot is drinking except me and I think I'm jealous. I'll be there as soon as they take down the barricades. And I'm very thirsty."

"So let's make her some iced tea, huh, Eve? Maybe lace it with some lemonade. You always liked that combination, didn't you?"

Eve nods enthusiastically. Even she's excited today.

Cass arrives shortly thereafter. As soon as we're seated out on the deck, she comments on how Eve seems so much brighter and sharper since the last time she visited. That's all I need to hear to make my day. As the midday sun shines down and the lake breeze tousles our "dos," we're all stifling yawns.

"Let's take catnaps now," I say, "then we can head on down to the Yum-Yum Tree for double-dip cones. I think that'll make a fine appetizer for the barbecued ribs for dinner. Don't you agree, Eve?"

She's just beaming, not necessarily in response to my plan.

After stuffing ourselves silly at dinner, we don jackets for the cool night to come and head for the backyard. All along the lakefront, tourists are sprouting in little groups, jockeying for position for the late-evening fireworks show on the harbor waters. And we have the best seats in the house.

Long about February, our town starts planning this lavish gift to locals and tourists. According to the town gossips, some really rich guy on the other side of the harbor donates the seed money for the fireworks display. All the townspeople, however, get into the act at the big winter fireworks fundraiser. One buck buys an "ooh," five bucks buys an "ahh," and ten bucks gets you a "WOW!" with an exclamation point. Due to circumstances beyond my control, we could only contribute a lowly "ooh" this year, but now we're filled with pride, just the same.

We set up our lawn chairs on our little beach bluff. While I divvy up some multicolored sparklers, a couple of tourist families wander into our backyard, with hopeful tentative smiles on their faces. Cass calls out, "Make yourselves at home, folks." Really, Cass.

And then the oohs, ahhs, and wows! begin. I'm a little concerned that the resounding ka-booms will rattle Eve. But no worry there. She's grabbing for a fresh sparkler before the other one burns out, lighting it, and simultaneously stuffing Yum-Yum Tree fudge in her mouth as fast and furiously as we are.

"Wow!" she says with her mouth full, then sips some lemonade.

What a night!

The next morning we all wander into the dining room a little hung over from yesterday's excitement. Yep, we alcoholics still manage to overdo things, with or without the booze. Cass wants to head back to Chicago late afternoon. But first, I suggest a picnic lunch at

Cave Point Park. Cass has never been there, and it's my favorite scenic spot and painting subject. Compared with California's Big Sur, Cave Point is anticlimactic. But we Midwesterners get a big kick out of any kind of rocky bluffs. Add some crashing waves and we've got a spellbinding spectacle of nature. It can enthrall me for hours.

I haven't trusted myself to take Eve there since the aneurysm. A person can break his neck pretty easily with one slip on the ever-moist rocky ledges. But Cass's presence emboldens me to suggest the field trip . . . and off we go.

This time of year, Cave Point's waves are relatively mellow. Still, they make loud swooshing and crashing sounds that set me atingle with anticipation for the next big wave heading in to the rocky shore.

Despite the posted warnings, several underage drinkers are jumping off the bluff into the hazardous waters below. I close my eyes to that sight. Too scary for me. We head on down the path, tripping over tree roots, until we reach a relatively secluded area. I can't resist taking a few photographs for my art source material, even though, at last count, I had 160 pictures of the area. I step out on the comparatively safe ledge, mindful of my own mild fear of heights, and beckon the always-bold Eve to follow. Surprisingly, she hangs back, holding on to white-faced Cass, who's clinging to a cedar tree.

"Why, Cass, I never knew you were afraid of heights." Wide-eyed, Cass just nods her head. "And how about you, Eve?" She nods, too. Well, son of a gun, somehow her subconscious has warned her about her balance problems.

"It's okay, Eve. I'm not going to force you," I say, as I retreat from the ledge. "And Cass, why didn't you mention your fear of heights when I described this place?"

She says, "I couldn't believe that rocky cliffs actually existed anywhere within 500 miles of Chicago." Now she has me laughing. Tourists!

The day after, and I'm feeling a big-time letdown from the little bit of excitement we managed to generate for the holiday. I'm also running late on paying the monthly bills. I have a sneaking suspicion I know why.

Whenever this old brain of mine starts acting spacey, it's because I'm procrastinating. So, what's to procrastinate? Aren't our days as uneventful as they can be?

Maybe now. But there's the small matter of how we're going to afford to continue living in our lakefront dream house. There's a short-term mortgage hanging over our heads and no way to start paying it back in the foreseeable future. I'm still a 24/7 caregiver here.

Anyway, I promised myself way back in January that I would come up with a strategy for dealing with this financial mess by July. Technically speaking, "by July" has passed. We're six days into the month and no plan has visited me, nor have I won the lottery. What shall I do?

"Do what you love and the money will follow." I can't tell you how many times that catchy classic book title pops into my brain and pretends to be *the* solution for all my problems. Maybe if I had a nice fat savings account, that strategy would work. But it's too risky now.

Guess I better sit down and do some serious brainstorming with myself. I bring out my trusty legal pad, some colored pens, and iced tea. Then I light a cigarette and I'm all set. Come on, subconscious, let's go!

Hmm . . . wait a second. Before I get going, better say a quick prayer. "God, grant me the serenity to accept the things I cannot change, courage to change the things I can, and the wisdom to know the difference." Please, God, I need an extra serving of wisdom today.

Now I'm ready. Doodle. Doodle. Yawn. Maybe it's time for a nap. Don't you dare. Okay, no need to yell. Hmm. "Do what you love; the money will follow." SHUT UP! Come on, subconscious. This isn't a game. I'm dead serious. "And I wasn't playing a game," a little voice says. Okay, I'll go with that tack, if only to banish it from my brain, once and for all.

So what do I love, for crying out loud? That's a no-brainer. I want to do my art. And maybe sell it from my own home-based art gallery, right here on beautiful Lake Michigan in downtown Baileys Harbor.

There, I said it. Now go away. But the thought doesn't go away. Why? Because it's really a GREAT idea!

"Eve, come here. I want to talk with you. Hurry, I think I have a great idea."

Eve groans as she rises from her easy chair in the living room. Dutifully, she takes the seat to my right at the dining room table.

"Now, please, pay attention. Five minutes, ten minutes tops. Here's the idea. I've decided that by August 15, we're going to open up our own home-based art gallery."

"You're crazy," she says, shaking her head.

"Yes, I am. But that's beside the point. I'm pretty sure this house is zoned 'mixed commercial.' That means we can convert the living room, hallway, and maybe the side bedroom into a gallery. We can hire Steve, the handyman, to build a removable divider to separate the gallery from the dining room. We'll move the TV and furniture in here, and use that huge kitchen for the dining area. Then we'll hire an electrician to install track lighting.

"Of course, we need an outdoor sign, too. What do you think, Eve? $2,000, maybe $3,000 tops."

Eve looks at me doubtfully.

"Look," I say, "despite appearances, this is not my ego run amok. I know it's going to be late in the tourist season, but if I can open this year, it'll teach me something. Then I can use the winter to paint saleable art and we can stage a grand reopening next spring.

"Seriously, Eve, I don't know how else to make any money up here to pay off that mortgage. I've been out of advertising too long. I'd go back to Chicago in a heartbeat, but all my old work leads have dried up. I've tried to contact them. Nothing. Zilch. I'm afraid we're going to lose the house before I can sell it.

"The stock market has gone south since 9/11. Even if I have the stamina to take one of those two-bit tourist jobs, all the money is going to go for a sitter for you. I can't leave you alone that long. Do you understand?"

Unhappy, Eve nods her head.

Now back to my plan. "Of course, I need to do some more painting.

Starting tomorrow I'll begin a marathon painting session. I think 20 12x16's will do the trick. With taking time out to do the bills and manage the house, I should have them finished in a month. That comes out to a painting a day." I pause to digest my words. I am crazy. I can't paint that fast. But then, why let that stop me from trying?

"Here's the best part of the idea, Eve. If I use that wraparound canvas, there's no need to frame. See? That means you won't have to do that, and I won't have to pay somebody else."

Eve smiles and nods. Yeah, I'll bet that suits her just fine.

"Wait a second. What am I saying, Eve? Of course, you should do the framing. I could enlarge some of the millions of photos I've taken. There must be at least ten that could qualify as 'art.' We'll use them as filler, maybe hang them in the front hall. Yeah, you could frame those."

Eve is eyeing me suspiciously now. She understands well enough to know that I'm talking about work for her to do. There's that four-letter word again. Framing is work. It requires precise measuring, adding, subtracting, and dividing. It's tricky. That's why I hate doing it.

"So, Eve, do you remember how to use a ruler?"

Though she's shaking her head rather vigorously, I choose to ignore her.

"Of course you do. And if you don't, I'll teach you. We'll give it a try this afternoon. Why don't you take a nap, so you'll be fresh and ready to work?" I try hard to stifle a snicker, but it escapes.

Eve sighs, rolls her eyes, and rises to take her nap. She is not a happy camper. Good. She's having an emotional reaction of sorts.

While Eve naps, I ransack our library, searching for her how-to books on framing. Back in Sedona, Eve had taken a framing class and then, in a fit of enthusiasm, invested way too much money in equipment, for a beginner. When we returned to Chicago, Eve took a job as an apprentice in a frame shop for a few months until she got bored with the nine-to-five routine, but not necessarily the framing. When we moved to Door County, she set up a frame station in the back bedroom. That's as far as it went, but maybe it still holds some intrigue for her. It's certainly worth a shot.

Refreshed by her nap, Eve's all set to tackle her new framing project. I first determine that she has virtually no memory of the tools of the trade and their functions. I conduct a guided tour of the back bedroom, stopping along the way to re-teach her how to use a ruler, a T-square, double-sided tape, and (uh-oh) a mat knife. I'm so focused, I miss the hilarity of the moment—talk about the blind leading the blind!

Three hours later, we've got a framed photo. If I squint, I can tell it's a wee bit cockeyed. But squinting causes eye wrinkles. So why do it?

"This is very good, Eve. Not perfect, but pretty darned good. We'll try again tomorrow morning. Dinnertime now: Hamburger Helper tonight. Maybe you can help me."

"We just had Hamburger Helper," Eve complains.

My, oh my, a short-term memory coup. I ponder this as I forage through the refrigerator, looking for a different dinner.

"Hey, Eve, how about brats? We could cook them on the grill. Hmmm, maybe you could do them." I wonder, dare I push her this late in the day? I just have this feeling that something clicked in Eve's mind while she repeated the framing routine. I can't fathom how framing would help bring back her short-term memory relative to meals, but apparently her mind made some kind of leap. "So what do you say? Do you have enough energy to try grilling?"

"Yeah, let me try." Eve looks almost eager.

"Okay, I'll keep my mouth shut. Show me what you remember about grill preparation. Talk it through while you do it."

"First, I need charcoal. Where's the charcoal?"

Silently, I shrug. Eve stands there thinking, then heads for the utility room. That's where it is, all right. Eve hauls out our little charcoal bin. Then heads back.

"I need lighter fluid. And where's that thing?"

"What thing?" I don't know what she's talking about.

"You know." She draws a picture in the air with her hands.

"Matches?" I ask. Then it dawns on me. "Oh, you mean that fancy push-button barbeque lighter."

"Never mind, I found it," Eve calls out from the utility room.

Good for her. I had no clue where it was.

Now we're out in the backyard with the grill. I stop the action so we can both take three deep breaths and relax. No expectations, I remind myself.

"Go for it, Eve."

Moving slowly, but with determination, Eve piles the briquettes into a little pyramid. Then she douses them with lighter fluid.

"Now pay attention, Eve," I interrupt. "Anytime you are around fire, please watch what you're doing."

With my warning, I assume her next actions will be tentative. Wrong. She goes for that lighter like she's drawing a gun. Before I can close my eyes—POOF—Eve makes fire. Luckily, it's okay. Only the charcoal is flaming, not us.

I breathe a sigh of relief. I actually broke a sweat on that one. Calm down. Act natural. Let Eve proceed.

And she does. Eve even insists on setting the table and chopping some onion. Yippee. Maybe Eve will rediscover the kitchen again.

That day comes sooner rather than later. One night, I am paying more attention to what Eve is doing rummaging through the refrigerator than to what I am doing at the stove.

"Uh-oh," I exclaim aloud.

"What's the matter?" Eve asks.

"I dumped the mushroom soup into the pan before I browned the chicken breasts. I've ruined our dinner."

"Oh, that's no problem," Eve responds. "Here, I'll fix it." She staggers over to the stove.

"What can you do?" I ask, not daring to hope that she has a solution.

"Out of my way," she commands me, as so many other "real," domesticated women have instructed me in the past. "Go see what's on TV tonight."

"Well, aren't we the little snot?" I automatically react defensively to the implication that I'm "less than" in the kitchen.

But, okay, I retreat and leave her alone to clean up my mess, not realizing what has taken place here until we're sitting down devouring a pretty decent dinner.

"Hey, Eve, did you notice? You're a cook again."

"Uh-huh," Eve says between bites.

"Guess you'll want to do it again tomorrow?"

"Uh-huh."

"Hmm. Maybe we better call Cass after dinner. You can talk about cooking with her. Does that sound like a good idea?"

"Uh-huh."

"Okay. Then I guess you can have your kitchen back."

"Thanks." Eve smiles knowingly.

That evening, I can feel the relaxation coursing through my body like a dip in a hot tub. Yeah, right, no expectations or hope for miracles. Unbeknownst to me, I must have been harboring a few expectations. Why else would I feel so relieved?

Since I'm on a roll, it may be a good time to revisit my plan for the home-based art gallery. Perhaps I can refine it or, better yet, realize the folly of it all and save myself from a lot of hard work and disappointment.

I retrieve my legal pad buried under the batch of today's bills. I'll just make a few notes to give my subconscious something to munch on while I sleep tonight.

The next morning, I awaken to a chorus of songbirds greeting the predawn light. I look at the clock. Geez, it's early. What's up with the birds, for Pete's sake? Looking outside, I see what the commotion is about. It looks like I woke up on another planet. Somebody painted the lake magenta. It's awesome.

I'm hypnotized by the light drama. Magenta waves are gently rolling in under a sherbet-striped sky. I can't believe the color play. This is the Midwest. Of course, there are the usual corals, pinks, and oranges at the horizon line. But above that are stripes of lemon yellow, lime green, and Colorado turquoise blue, punctuated by rose-tipped, dark magenta clouds.

But I am so sleepy, I nod off again. When I awaken at seven, I wonder if it was a dream—or a hallucination—or a sign from the Almighty. I'll never know. I didn't take a picture.

At breakfast, I give up trying to describe the dawn's early light to Eve. Even my subconscious can't relate to a lemon-lime sky and fuchsia lake. When Eve toddles off to get dressed, I do a mental check to see if there are any intuitive thoughts about the gallery running around in my head. Nope. Oh, well, time for meditation anyway. I grab my pile of spiritual daily reading material.

Just as I'm opening the first book, a tiny voice trumpets in my head: "If you convert the living room into a gallery, it will help you sell the house. You can distract attention from all the defects this old house has to offer." In other words, it's my chance to make some lemonade out of this lemon.

I go with it. I certainly don't need a Realtor to tell me our house lacks "curb appeal." Anybody can see we don't have a curb. Though our front view is blissfully camouflaged by a stand of cedars, prospective buyers still have to walk up a long potholed driveway that we share with the auto-repair garage next door. I know I appreciate the convenience of an on-premise car mechanic, but I am not sure others will. If I install a big attention-attracting gallery sign at the end of the driveway, however, it could give prospects something more interesting to focus on as they walk up to the house.

Another gallery sign on the front door will solve our confusing front-door situation. We have two. One leads to the utility room; the other opens on a long, dark hallway leading to the living room. It's not very inviting right now. But with a gallery, I have an excuse to install track lighting and line the hall walls with my photographs. Once in the living room, I presume the lake view will capture anyone's attention—that is, if the prospects don't trip on our threadbare carpeting. After living with that pukey pinky-beige carpet for two years, the thought of recarpeting just to sell a house plays havoc with my serenity.

With the "store décor," however, I can cover the threadbare spots with area mats or counter displays. Minus the big furniture, I will have all the design flexibility I need to redirect the eye. Plus the necessary track lighting for the painting display in the living room will be a real sales feature for the house. After seeing that room first, the prospects will be so discombobulated they won't notice that our house is actually a duplex built piecemeal over the decades. Maybe I can solve a $10,000 fix-up problem with a $2,000 investment.

I phone my Chicago friends, Roger and Merle, to ask their opinion on my idea. Roger grumbles that it's about time I put the house up for sale. That means he approves the idea. Merle is so enthusiastic, she volunteers to come and ready the house for market. I quickly hang up after accepting her offer; I don't want to give her time to change her mind. I sure could use the help . . . or at least some handholding and maybe an evening out.

Later that morning, Eve and I review our framing lessons from yesterday and try again. This time I hand her the mat, picture, and frame without instructions. I encourage her to organize her tools, wanting her to develop a rhythm—no matter how slow she actually works. I ask her to "teach" me what she's doing. In framing, in the 12-Step program, in rehabilitation, in day-to-day life, I believe we learn best by teaching our experience, skills, and knowledge to another. In half the time it took us yesterday, we finish another project.

Both of us are surprised by the excellent result. Once again, doing the action has helped Eve remember not only the general principles of her task, but also some obscure tricks of the trade. Now if I can just get her to converse with me more.

Another week passes. I'm painting from morning until night with varying results. Eve spends two to three hours a day in her framing room with the door closed. She tells me she's framing, but I haven't seen anything yet.

Eve ends the suspense one bright summer morn. "Da da da dah!" she heralds her own arrival in the dining room, where I've taken a painting break to do bills. She's holding two framed photos.

"Very nice, very professional, Eve." While I'm admiring her work, she brings out three more. "Wow. You're becoming a regular speed demon. Nice work, Eve."

"I also have a surprise for you," she announces.

Oooh, that makes me nervous, but I say, "Okay, surprise me."

Eve disappears, and then returns holding what is obviously one of my pastel paintings, beautifully framed. I'm stunned. Tears fill my eyes.

Of all the major art media, pastel is perhaps the most difficult to frame. In her pre-aneurysm days, Eve would curse the medium. Not only does it smear easily, I complicate it by never allowing enough margin to grip the painting properly. Pastels are always framed under antistatic glass with spacer bars to keep the painting away from the glass. I have never attempted to frame one of my own pastels.

And there's Eve, standing there with this big smile on her face, showing off a beautiful framing job.

"Why, Eve, what a wonderful belated Thanksgiving-Christmas-Easter-birthday gift. That's worth a huge hug and a kiss."

She's so proud of herself and I'm simply awed. That's a miracle, all right.

The next week Merle arrives with Margie, a mutual A.A. acquaintance, in tow. In her inimitable style, Merle announces that it's time for all of us to get this house in shape for a sale. And, by the way, she's in charge.

Thanks to Merle and Margie, the utility room (our foyer) receives a major facelift with a fresh coat of paint and new indoor-outdoor carpeting. Flexing our female muscles in unison, we are able to relocate the big pieces of furniture from the living room to the dining room. Plus generous Merle treats all of us to a couple of evenings with the tourists—a fish boil and a dinner theater at a local supper club. Ah, yes, the performing arts are alive and thriving in summertime Door. I've been so focused on the drama at home that the concept of escape by buying into fictional drama can hardly hold my attention. What man-made plot can compare to grocery shopping at Piggly Wiggly with Eve?

Merle and Margie have done all they can. The rest is up to us.

The next day it's back to our daily marathon painting and framing sessions. One morning I take a time-out to check in with Eve's rehab doctor.

Yes, Eve seems to be focusing better without the drugs designed to help her do that. And, thanks to a rigid bi-hourly bathroom routine, Eve is managing to stay mostly dry during the day. Nighttime continence presents another problem. Since February, I have been forcing myself to stay awake until midnight, so I can awaken Eve for a potty visit. It's always a crap shoot whether she'll be dry at that time, or if she'll stay dry throughout the night. She continues to have no awareness of signals for most bodily functions, including blowing her nose or clearing her throat.

"I can prescribe a pill for nighttime continence," the doctor offers.

What? There's a pill for that? Where has this man been? Doesn't he listen? I've been losing sleep and changing sheets daily for months, and now he tells me there's a pill. I want to throttle him— but not until he calls in the prescription.

By the end of the week, my feeling of frustration is trumped by utter joy. Eve's been dry for three nights running. It's such a tiny pill it will get lost on the altar I want to build for it.

Every day after breakfast, I ask Eve to read to me from two or three of our A.A. daily meditation books and to summarize the messages. Then I conduct a short subconscious cheerleading exercise. After the one-to-ten relaxation count, I implore the subconscious to stay open to the creative spirit we will need for our painting and framing tasks. I ask it to help us remember the techniques we've learned in the past so we can work more efficiently. I remind it that our motivation for opening this gallery is to be able to afford our beautiful view of the lake and harbor, or if that's not possible, to use the gallery to attract a potential home buyer.

Either way, our goal is to have the gallery open for this year's tourist season. Finally, I ask for help for Eve to use the framing and gallery preparation process to help her increase her awareness, improve her ability to focus, and sharpen her memory of how to apply those skills. With that, I count backward, asking for enthusiasm and energy along the way. As always, I say a prayer, asking God for help in aligning my will with His and telling Him that I trust that whatever happens will be okay. Some days I believe my prayer, some days I don't, but I say it anyway.

By Labor Day weekend—way beyond my deadline—we open our gallery doors. The photos aren't bad and my paintings are passable. But already my focus has switched to selling the house.

Outside, a steady drizzle ensures that potential gallery customers will stay away in droves. I have no illusions about the drawing power of my outdoor gallery shop sign; I just pray it'll do its job of distracting attention from the ugly approach to our now "For Sale" lake house.

I'm seated in a cozy chair in the corner of our living room gallery, waiting to hear the tinkle of the entry bells. I note that we've done a pretty good job of camouflaging the flaws in the carpeting. The rain has picked up, transforming my beloved lake view into a blur of silvery grays. By contrast, our new track lighting brightens the room considerably.

In fact, the redesign of the interior is probably the best example of real art in the living room. For some reason, I find this thought highly amusing. Here I am in the middle of my lifetime dream, the proprietor of a home-based art gallery on the Door shore of Lake Michigan. I want to cry. Instead, I fall asleep.

"Donna, wake up. Your shift is over. My turn." Eve's shaking my shoulder. "I made a baloney sandwich and a cup of tea for you. They're on the dining room table."

Now *that* is the highlight for this day.

In the days before the gallery opening, I gave Eve a crash course in customer relations, counting money, calculating tax. On day two of the Labor Day weekend, she declares that she will manage the gallery while I pay the bills and paint some more.

It's sunny outside, which usually guarantees that tourists will want to come inside to entertain themselves. Go figure. Anyway, I finally hear the tinkle of the bells, heralding our first prospect. I wish I had a medal to reward the customer's bravery. I'm all ears as I tune in to Eve's first attempt at bantering with customers. Not bad, Eve. Even brain-damaged, Eve is a "natural" with people. Too quickly I hear the bells again, indicating the customer's hasty retreat.

"Hey, Eve," I call out. "What scared her off? Did you belch or snort at her?"

"Naw. I think it was the $400 price tag on your sailboat painting," Eve retaliates.

And so the day progresses. Along about three o'clock, our little bells go crazy. My goodness, three customers at once! I decide I'd better join Eve, though I'm not sure there will be room for all of us. As I make my entrance, I almost knock over the trifold screen that separates the gallery from the dining room and our curious cats.

"Welcome," I greet the couple staring at me as I catch the screen and shoo the cats away. "Don't mind me. Feel free to browse."

"Uh, okay," the guy replies. "But actually we came in to look at the house. The sign says it's for sale, right?"

Oh, my God! I can't believe what I'm hearing. My idea actually worked. We caught ourselves a real estate prospect.

I'm totally flustered. The house isn't officially on the market yet. And where's my Realtor? On a family picnic, I think. What to do? The rest of the house is a disaster. Clean, but it's a mess. I don't think I hung up my pajamas. Lordy.

"Sure, I'll show you the house," I say, "but be forewarned, I wasn't expecting to show it until Tuesday."

"That's okay," he smiles broadly. "We're up from Milwaukee. Going back tomorrow. We'd sure appreciate your showing it to us. Do you have a listing sheet?"

"Sure, come on into the dining room." I struggle once more with the flimsy screen and the cats. "Lola, Ozzie, out of my way. Hope you're not allergic to cats. This dining room is a mess. I think you'll really like the view from the master bedroom." Uh-oh. Nervous motor mouth is off and running. Shut up, Donna!

I toss the papers helter-skelter, looking for the listing photocopies. I find one, hand it to him, and hold my breath. I'm asking big bucks for this disaster.

He looks it over, nudges his wife and smiles. So, okay, what's big bucks to me is actually a bargain for the financially solvent select of the world.

By the end of the week, we have an offer; in two more weeks, we have a deal.

# 20

# Pass It On

It's only two months from the contract to closing on our home, but most of the days are filled with enough incidents of ineptitude and sneaky maneuverings to make it the real estate transaction from hell. Welcome back to the real world, Donna.

Of course, selling the house creates another hairy problem. Where are we moving to? I have no idea. A quick online check of the suburban Chicago real estate scene tells me the best "view" we can afford is that of a parking lot from the window of a too-small condominium. Needless to say, we can't afford a view of a cow barn in northern Door either.

I try to involve Eve in the decision-making process, but it's difficult to interpret her minimalist emotional reactions to my suggestions. I am well aware that her life savings are at stake, so I'm constantly on the phone with my sponsor, checking my motivations.

We embark on a quick house-hunting trip to the Madison area, where I might have a chance of landing a Wisconsin university or government job. Sadly, the experience confirms my suspicion that real estate values "down south" have skyrocketed. On the plus side, I think I'm finally cured of my false belief that a geographic change will ever solve my problems.

One evening, while I am trying to bury my house-hunting woes with butter pecan ice cream, smothered with hot fudge sauce, Eve speaks.

"Why haven't we looked in Sturgeon Bay?" she asks. "Aren't there lots of cute little houses in town? We came up here because your dream was Door County. Sturgeon Bay is the center. I want to look there."

Okey-dokey. Eve has spoken.

Within a week, we make an offer on a renovated Cape Cod near downtown Sturgeon Bay. It's accepted. Hard to complain when both Lake Michigan and Green Bay are only a mile or so away and it's five blocks to the connecting canal. The walk will do us good.

Meanwhile, I'm packing as fast as I can. I forgive myself for my out-of-control knickknack collection and overabundance of art supplies, but Eve takes it on the chin for the hundreds of books in her library. I must admit that my regular relaxation routine has flown the coop these days. Too bad, because between the real estate debacle and the pandemonium of packing, we both could use a little more serenity.

It's time for Eve to learn a new occupational therapy exercise. "Please," I say, "I'm begging you to pay attention to me, Eve. I desperately need your help to meet the closing date. This is packing tape. These are dangerous scissors. And those are folded boxes. Now I will demonstrate how you used to put together boxes. Actually, you were rather anal about it, but I'll pop for all the extra tape your method requires. Okay? Watch me do one, then it's your turn."

Somewhere, in the back of my mind, there's a nagging thought that professional therapists would frown on my involving Eve in the chaos of packing. I'm sorry that I have to introduce Eve to the concept of survival at this stage in her life, but that's the way the cookie crumbles.

"Okey-dokey. Next we're going to play hide-and-seek. Every hour or so, you'll check on me, wherever in this house I'm packing. You'll look for filled boxes with a piece of notepaper on top. Those are the ones you will seal with tape and mark accordingly. I doubt I'll have time to double-check you, so remember that whatever labeling mistakes you make, we'll have to live with them when we unpack. Got it? Good. Let's go."

Now we're clicking, even making good progress. I contact the only moving company in town. They offer some suggestions on how we can cut corners in packing, but of course it costs us dearly in moving expenses. It doesn't matter; I just want out.

By December 10, we're in our cute little house with the big beautiful basement for storage. By December 11, I've unpacked the kitchen and arranged it as best as I can. It's the way Eve likes it, I hope. I push myself to fill the curio cabinet in the living room to display our favorite knickknacks. After hanging seven paintings on the bare living area walls, I call it "home, sweet home" and take a break for the holidays.

"I'll finish unpacking after Christmas. It's December 17 and we need a Christmas tree."

"Who cares about a tree?" Eve comments and shrugs.

Ohhh, now that makes me mad. "I do, dammit. And you better. I don't care if you can't feel your emotions. You're going to start acting as if you can. Christmas may not be your favorite holiday, but once upon a time it was mine.

"Don't you dare forget I spent last Christmas Eve by myself in a hotel, then said hi to Santa in the hospital Christmas morning, and watched him give you—not me—presents. We're not only going hunting for a Christmas tree today, I'm going to take you shopping for me. Here's 20 bucks. You will surprise me with a Christmas gift, and we're going to have fun—or else. Do I make myself clear?"

"Perfectly," Eve reluctantly replies.

"Now get dressed in several layers. I don't want to hear any moaning that you're cold while we're shopping for a tree, or that you're too hot when we're in the store. And smile, dammit."

Eve forces a toothy smile. Nevertheless, I think she gets the message. I am a caregiver at the end of my rope. I believe even God feels sorry for me, because after visiting two empty Christmas tree lots, we serendipitously find the last pre-cut Christmas tree in town.

Yessiree. After driving around in circles for an hour, we come upon a makeshift tree lot at an abandoned gas station. The shivering proprietor switches his attention away from a portable TV long enough to say, "You can have that tree leaning against the truck for five bucks. Then I can go home and have a couple of shots while I watch the Packers game. Brrr, it's cold."

"There, Eve, you can be grateful we found a pre-cut Christmas tree," I say, as I drive away. "No telling what would have happened had I been forced to go into the forest with you to chop down my own tree with my sharp little axe."

Eve gives me the eye, not certain if I really mean what I say. Let her wonder.

Once I get the Christmas lights and ornaments on the tree—I wouldn't call it "decorating"—my sense of serenity starts to return. For the next week, I allow myself to do absolutely nothing except buy groceries, eat them, and watch over Eve.

A day or two before Christmas, I discover several packs of Christmas cards in a box. I decide to get in the spirit by writing thank-you notes to everyone who helped us over the past year. It's amazing how this simple action of gratitude helps me reclaim my sanity and more serenity.

For me, Christmas Eve is the most enchanting night of the year. Long gone is the Czechoslovakian family celebration at my Auntie Marie's house on "Candy Cane Lane" in Chicago. No matter. Thanks to my overactive imagination and visual mind, I can relive the tummy-tingling excitement of yesteryear anywhere, anytime.

Over morning coffee, I entertain Eve and me with my vivid memories of Christmases past. "Then, we'd all rise to say grace before dinner. Dad would lead the prayer, followed by a little prayer in Czechoslovakian. He could never remember the words, so Auntie Irene would help him. What made it more fun was the lights would be turned off, as he said, 'Corners, my dear little corners. God bless the corners of this house.' Then he'd throw walnuts over his shoulder into the corners. We kids would duck, then run to the corners where a silver dollar would be waiting for each of us."

Eve chimes in, "In my house it was the Polish custom to share oplatki before dinner. That's wafer bread, you know."

"Yeah, we had it, too. With honey, as I recall. Weren't those meat-less meals fabulous? I haven't tasted fish like that since. I think my aunties would go down to the Fulton Street market to buy it fresh. How about your mom, Eve? Hey, wait a second. Isn't there a great fish market in Algoma? Since we moved, it's only 20 minutes away. Come on, Eve, let's go see what we can find for dinner. We can continue reminiscing in the car."

We return from Algoma with smoked fish and frozen shrimp. It's what Eve says she feels comfortable in preparing. Later, while I'm lining up the Christmas CD playlist for the evening, I notice Eve is ransacking the cupboards.

"Here they are," she announces with glee. I look up as Eve emerges with a plastic container of ugly brown things.

"Here are what?" I ask her.

"My dried Polish mushrooms. I'm going to make the traditional Polish sweet-sour mushroom soup for dinner."

"Isn't that really complicated, Eve? Did you find the recipe?"

"Yep. But I think I can use this canned beef stock to shortcut the process."

With that, my serenity flies out the window. Eve's guardian angel and I fight for position as I hover over Eve during the soup-cooking process. But there's no need to worry. It's obvious Eve knows what she's doing, as she elbows me out of the way.

Her eyes are as bright and shiny as that famous star when we finally sit down to dinner. It's a Christmas celebration I never could have imagined one short year ago . . . and one of those presents that money can't buy.

As the year draws to an end, Eve receives a surprise check from the Veteran's Administration. It's been only 13 months since I filed the claim. Anyway, they announce that Eve qualifies for compensation as the disabled widow of a veteran. So, pooh on you, Social Security. We're going to make it without you.

Though the influx of cash solves some immediate problems, I figure it will keep the wolves from the door for only a couple of years. By then, Eve will qualify for Social Security's regular widow's benefit. But what about me? I'm living off her, still trapped by her need for 24/7 supervision. I don't have to worry about a job until late spring, however, because there are none.

Maybe now's the time to write that book . . . perhaps an account of the aneurysm story. Maybe make it a mystery. It's an idea. I'll start outlining in January.

So I do. It keeps my mind out of the "poor me's" all winter long. Meanwhile, Eve is assuming responsibility for all meal preparation and grocery shopping. I go along to give her a ride.

Despite the challenge of Wisconsin winters, Eve is walking daily. As winter melts into spring, I notice she's more coordinated, less robotic in her arm swings. In addition, she's turning her head left and right while she walks. I encourage it by asking for a play-by-play of what she visually perceives as we walk.

One fine April day, I bite the bullet and suggest we go for a car ride. Eve's been vicariously driving from the shotgun position for several months now, pretending to brake, accelerate, steer, and turn when I do. But this time, I tell her she can drive for real. And do you know what? She can! In this, I can barely tell the difference between the old Eve and the new Eve. My good sense tells me not to test her skills on a high-speed highway, but all systems are "go" for driving around town.

It's also time for us to return to A.A. meetings on a regular basis. I decide we'll try the one all-women's meeting in town. Happily, several of the women have significant sobriety and, more important, the patience to listen to Eve as she tries to express herself through the fog of long- and short-term memory loss, mental confusion, and lack of practice speaking in public. The encouragement of strangers does wonders for Eve's confidence and conversational skills.

During the summer, we return to NEW for several psychological therapy sessions as Eve continues to search for her ever-elusive emotions.

Brain, Heal Thyself

As Eve improves, I'm beginning to see more clearly the challenges that lie ahead for her. Always happy-go-lucky, Eve will have to dig deep for the motivation to continue her recovery. She resists a daily routine and my suggestions even to try. When Eve is bored, her first impulse is to read, her second is to play on the computer. Ever the addictive personality—with or without alcohol—Eve gets a "high" by sneaking in a computer solitaire game or two.

I feel more frustration than I ever have during this rehabilitation period. Obviously, I *expected* at some point that Eve would want to work to improve her mind. I find myself tiptoeing along a too-thin line, teetering between caregiving/rehabilitation and enabling. It's making me nuts enough that my sponsor insists I read Al-Anon's codependency-oriented daily meditations.

Three years after the brain aneurysm, Eve continues to improve, thereby debunking the professionally proffered prediction that there's only a two-year window for recovery.

Though I am still not comfortable leaving her alone on my rare overnight trips, she usually does okay while I am at work on my part-time job. As long as she avoids the pitfalls of reading or computer play during the day, she stays alert until 8 P.M. This I know from watching her participate in two evening A.A. meetings per week.

A writer in her own right in those pre-aneurysm days, Eve is typing every word of this book and helping me edit it. Every day we argue over her desire to replace my beloved dashes with her more formal semicolons and commas. In my humble, nonprofessional estimation, Eve has recovered 90 percent of her faculties.

We don't *expect* that 100-percent recovery is possible, but we do continue *to act as if* it is. As the 12-Step program suggests, we simply continue trying to do the next right thing, turning the results over to the care of our Higher Power. It's a "we" program, you know.

# 21

# Commentary by
# Lawrence J. Beuret, M.D.

The medical literature has documented the role of the subconscious mind in curing illnesses as trivial as the common cold and as deadly as metastatic tumors. To my knowledge, however, this is the first anecdotal report on the enlistment of the subconscious in reversing the devastating effects of a brain aneurysm, stroke, and seizures.

When the medical community encounters a recovery that runs contrary to all expectation, it's common to suggest a faulty diagnosis, but in Eve's case, this explanation simply won't work. She did suffer a ruptured aneurysm; parts of her functional brain were destroyed. When medical treatment and professional rehabilitation had done all they could, Donna was left with two clear choices: accept the permanence of her friend's impaired function, or devise some way to rescue Eve from her state of nearly total dependency. Fortunately, Donna chose the latter course.

In her daily rehabilitation program for Eve, Donna recognized and creatively applied these two short rules of the subconscious mind: The subconscious always works to ensure an individual's physical and spiritual survival; and the subconscious is most receptive to emotionally laden appeals for assistance in fulfilling its primal role as protector of the self.

In its broadest terms, Eve's recovery was based on two factors. The first was the unique way the brain stores and retrieves information, and the second was the equally unique way in which the subconscious can be stimulated to retrieve previously stored memories. Still, this leaves unexplained how an injured brain can regain the memories it has lost through traumatic injury.

Historically, there have been two different ways to explain how the brain stores memories and information.

In the 1920s, research with rats demonstrated that no matter how much of the brain was removed, the rat still "remembered" how to perform complex tasks learned prior to the surgery. This suggested that memory might not be located in specific locations, but generalized throughout the brain.

Later research performed during brain surgery on human patients showed that electrical stimulation of certain areas of the brain's temporal region retrieved specific memories. These experiments seemed to indicate that individual memories existed only in specific areas of the brain. Destroy one of those areas, the reasoning went, and its information would be destroyed as well.

This theory quickly gained favor with the scientific community. After all, it's more palatable to compare human brains with other human brains than to suggest a similarity between human beings and rats. For all its popularity, however, the "specific region–specific memory" theory failed to explain how patients could recover from strokes that had destroyed portions of the brain.

In the 1960s, research by Stanford University's Karl Pribram suggested that memory was like a hologram. (A hologram is a laser image, the entirety of which can be retrieved from any of its fragments.) Pribram concluded that the earlier research on rats was valid and that human memory, instead of being localized in specific cells, was generalized throughout the brain.

Generalized memory gives the brain two powerful advantages: It can store more memories; and if the brain is damaged, its stored memories will be less susceptible to destruction.

This explains how Eve was able to recover so much of her brain function and memory: Donna's intuition, coupled with her knowledge of how the conscious and subconscious interact, helped Eve tap into her holographically stored memories.

Throughout her narrative, Donna describes how Eve's recovery did not progress gradually and evenly, but by astonishing leaps, as if masses of connections were being restored at one time. This "leaps and bounds" progress powerfully supports the holographic theory.

Still the question remains: What part did Eve's subconscious play in this recovery, and how was Donna able to help her employ it?

Thanks to her years of experience in advertising and her fascination with visualization techniques, Donna understood the theory and practice of interaction between the conscious and subconscious mind. This understanding enabled Donna to turn daily interactions with Eve into therapeutic tools that shaped her recovery.

As Donna knew, the conscious mind and the subconscious mind relate to one another as a logical, or linear, thinker and a creative, or divergent, thinker might do. When two such personalities interact, the linear thinker might wonder, "Where on earth is she coming from? Why doesn't she stay on the subject? What does that observation have to do with anything?" The creative thinker, on the other hand, might perceive the logician as cold, judgmental, boring, and lacking in sympathy.

Conscious thinking is linear, logical, and language-based. Subconscious thinking derives from clusters of memories and emotions connected by association. It is branching and nonlinear, and, to the linear thinker, appears random and chaotic.

## Comparative Functions

| | Subconscious | Conscious |
|---|---|---|
| Operational System | Beliefs | Factual knowledge; Logic |
| Action | Store; Protect; Ensure survival | Filter; Analyze; Judge; Construct |
| Access | Imagery; Dreams; Altered states: Reduced consciousness, Free association, Brainstorming, Hypnosis | Conscious thinking; Conscious awareness |
| Connections | Association: Time, Place; Similarity of: Emotion, Feeling, Sensory stimulus, Physical sensation; Nonlinear; Symbolic; Literal | Abstract; Chrono-logical; Logical; Linear; Language based |
| Expression | Verbal slips; Semantic inconsistencies; Involuntary thought; Involuntary movement; Nonverbal responses; Body language; Imagery; Dreams | Verbal; Conscious thought; Voluntary movement; Language |

For the reader who only wants to know *why* the techniques Donna employed had worked, the table of **Comparative Functions** is designed to provide this insight in a very compact and summarized format. By her intuitive choice of imagery as the vehicle for communication with Eve's subconscious, Donna has employed the most efficient and the most global approach available. The table of **Comparative Functions** illustrates the polar opposition of functions of these two areas of the mind. Each has its strengths, but each has its shortcomings. Only a clear understanding of both minds will allow one to avoid the pitfalls associated with trying to apply the processes of one mind to the other. A logical, linear, and rational approach to convincing the brain that it had the ability to heal itself would have had no effect on a conscious mind that was intermittently and only marginally operational. Likewise, as Eve began to regain higher-level conscious functions, allowing her to wallow in the realm of the undisciplined associative processes of the subconscious would have contributed nothing to her eventual regaining of her former intellectual abilities.

The process of brainstorming illustrates perfectly how the conscious and subconscious interact.

The purpose of brainstorming is the production of ideas—any ideas. They needn't be connected; they needn't even appear to be relevant. The logical mind is horrified by brainstorming, judging it a waste of time. Once the brainstorming process is well under way, however, information can move in and out of the subconscious with equal facility, generating ideas and solutions that the conscious mind, with its rigid and judgmental cast, could never conceive of. Brainstorming works well, as long as the logical mind does not interfere and begin eliminating ideas on the basis of their "relevance" or "usefulness."

As Donna understood, subconscious associations can generate countless connections through emotions, sensual experiences, physical sensations, and proximity of time. These connections, and Donna's understanding of how to encourage them, enabled Eve to reconnect to the memories and skills that had comprised so much of her former self.

On the face of it, a comatose state might seem ideal for establishing communication with the subconscious: After all, the conscious mind can scarcely be engaged when the patient is unconscious. Research suggests otherwise. Unimpeded access may occur from time to time, but apparently it is random and rare. The caregiver must therefore be alert for opportune moments when communication with the subconscious can be established.

Fortunately, Donna's knowledge and intuition told her when the subconscious was ready to communicate, and to be communicated with. While Eve is unconscious, Donna recognizes that her attempts at stimulation are largely useless. She learns to look for Eve's involuntary movements (e.g., a shift of position) or a nonverbal response (e.g., coughing) as signs that Eve's subconscious is ready to communicate, and to receive communication.

Another critical shift occurs when Donna realizes that her role has changed from caregiver ("babysitting a vegetable") to rehabilitator. She must become an observant detective, ready at a moment's notice to identify and utilize her infrequent opportunities for communication. This enables her to perform a role that no one else can fill, not even the medical and professional personnel who are involved in Eve's rehabilitation.

This shift was as important for caregiver as for patient: Suddenly Donna moved from a position of passive helplessness to one of proactive empowerment. It was at this critical point that Eve's recovery became possible.

Throughout Eve's recovery period, both in the hospital and at home, Donna's recognition of communications from Eve's subconscious became increasingly sensitive and sophisticated. As we have already seen, the subconscious employs two important ways to communicate: involuntary movement and nonverbal cues. Both require a caregiver's interpretation to give them context.

For example, when Donna recognizes the mischievous look that precedes Eve's placing the pegs in the "wrong" places, her interpretation of Eve's action is critical to the direction of her rehabilitation. If Eve is so damaged and retarded that she can no longer recognize simple shapes and colors, then she has become a vegetable, and further efforts at rehabilitation will do her little good. If, on the other hand, Eve is so bored with the elementary nature of the activity that she refuses to cooperate with it, it's logical to assume that Eve's mind (and her sense of humor!) are both intact, and, further, that there is every reason to expect a further degree of recovery.

Indirect suggestion (speaking of "when" something will happen when it hasn't yet happened at all) and expectation (the choosing of

# Commentary by Lawrence J. Beuret, M.D.

goals for others without their consent) offer two more ways to deal with the subconscious. At first glance, both of these methods might seem sure to succeed, because both eliminate the conscious mind from their application.

With indirect suggestion, this often holds true. The subconscious mind, no less than the conscious mind, prefers empowerment—the idea of being fully in charge of its choices. With expectation, success is less certain because the subconscious, like a willful child, resists being told directly what it should do. Unless applied with great subtlety and tact, expectation can arouse resentment in the subconscious, leading to the rejection of whatever goal the expectation was meant to achieve.

Donna's experiences with the A.A. 12-step program gave her a certain caution in working with Eve. It was vital, she realized, to step back and allow Eve to listen to her own subconscious cues. Donna herself would often sense that Eve was ready for another quantum leap and would be ready to assist her when the moment came to act.

A perfect example of this process was Eve's consent to go to the post office. Donna's intuition told her that Eve was too dependent on her to help her dress, and yet getting dressed was an obvious prerequisite for going to the post office. This, if you will, was an "imbedded" indirect suggestion: Donna was willing to let Eve struggle getting dressed because, by consenting to go to the post office, Eve had implicitly consented to the steps required to achieve it.

In this instance, Donna's intuition and the decision that followed it worked perfectly, setting Eve up for success—and, as it turned out, not merely for success, but for achievement well beyond her own expectations. Donna's common-sense reactions to Eve's subconscious cues would become a powerful tool in further awakening Eve's sense of self-reliance and self-worth.

Employing variations of imagery also contributed powerfully to Eve's eventual recovery. At the conclusion of Eve's final rehabilitation session, the unmistakable "professional" implication was: This is as good as Eve will ever get; don't waste your time trying to make her any better. But since Donna was unwilling to accept that assessment, the question facing her was "How do I proceed from here? How can I attempt to regain what Eve has lost?" Paradoxically, the answer was: You don't. Instead, you enlist the help of Eve's subconscious, the only ally that can help her now.

Yet another example of Donna's use of imagery was her visualizing shoveling paths through snow when she was struggling to find new ways to help Eve. That powerful image was all Donna's subconscious needed: It entered her subconscious, which obligingly came up with memories of the fishing game she used to play as a child. This, in turn, led to the idea of helping Eve "fish" for emotions.

Imagery and visualization would play a continuing role in other areas of Eve's rehabilitation. Maxwell Maltz related how the mental rehearsal of kinesthetic tasks—those requiring physical movements—developed or improved their efficiency in real life. Memories of finely tuned repetitive movement are retained in the cerebellum, a smaller part of the brain lying just below the larger cerebral hemispheres, the familiar left and right halves of the brain. The mental rehearsal Maltz prescribed appeared to develop and refine these kinesthetic pathways in the cerebellum.

Donna demonstrated Maltz's principles in the way she taught Eve to drive again. They would sit in the car and mentally rehearse, over and over again, all of the movements and tasks that driving required. Not surprisingly, Eve rapidly recovered the basic driving skills she once possessed. The return of Eve's cooking skills, a skill in which she also had always shown a keen interest, began to return at a remarkable rate.

The most dramatic return of kinesthetic memory was the revival of Eve's former picture matting and framing skills. By Donna's simply reacquainting her with the basics of using a ruler and matting knife, Eve was able to recover these skills independently in a matter of a few hours. That the relearning of this skill was critical to preventing the eventual loss of the house may certainly have been a major factor in Eve's subconscious motivation to reconnect with this skill.

Donna's narrative provides a detailed picture of what was happening, but little indication of how it was being accomplished. The answer may ultimately lie in the very characteristic of the subconscious that has kept it from being clearly identified and localized within the brain: its diffuseness and unwillingness to assign specific activities to specific regions of the brain. It may be this diffuse character of the subconscious that allowed it to escape the devastation experienced in more clearly identified areas of the conscious mind.

## The Caregiver

We have dealt at length with the stratagems a caregiver may use to help a brain-injured victim recover her former memories and skills. But what of the caregiver herself? What are her stresses and needs?

The long-term prospects for a brain-injured individual's recovery, once the basic medical and institutional rehabilitation processes have been completed, rest solely on the caregiver in the patient's home. Those who have had firsthand experience with this process may find that what follows is all too familiar. For an individual unfamiliar with the experience, however, it is important to appreciate the kind of disruption and personal stress a catastrophic medical emergency can bring about.

For a rough parallel, we can turn to the events of September 11, 2001. In one searing instant, an incomprehensible event turned an ordinary day into one of grief and horror. Thousands of persons who had started the day expecting it to be like any other were either killed outright or suddenly rendered unconscious and unresponsive, requiring immediate, lifesaving medical care. Just as with the 9/11 experience, the initial response to a family member's or friend's catastrophic injury might be one of unreality and disorientation: "This can't be happening to me." For some, the sudden role of caregiver may inspire energetic mobilization; for others, it may induce an overwhelming paralysis of the will. Regardless of the caregiver's initial reaction, however, the process of initial medical care involves a series of bewildering decisions that the new caregiver must make while still in a state of shock.

Donna's narrative gives firsthand insight into what it's like to be thrust suddenly into the role of caregiver without a moment's foreknowledge or preparation. Through the initial phases, when highly skilled medical personnel provide most of the care, the days involve long periods of anxious waiting interspersed with an urgent need to make decisions about totally unfamiliar matters. Family and friends offer positive support, but it may be accompanied with unwanted or unwelcome "stories" or irrelevant advice based on others' anxieties or personal experiences.

For caregivers to be most effective during the acute initial phase of the process, as well as in the chronic, long-term phase of institutional medical and rehabilitation processes, they must understand what is happening in their life. They must appreciate the "stresses" to which caregivers are commonly subject. To facilitate that understanding, I closely define the overused and vague term "stress" as "the need to confront unexpected changes in routine and normal daily function."

In the 1960s, there was a movement within the disciplines of medicine, psychiatry, and psychology to define exactly what stress was and how it could be quantified. The extensive research and writings of Hans Selye had provided great insight into how an individual or organism is affected by stress—for example, increased secretion of specific stress hormones. But this vast area of investigation failed to be able to define what constituted stress for individual persons, since what may constitute stress for one person may scarcely affect another.

In the 1970s, conferences explored the subject and tried to provide a scientific approach to subjective stress. One outcome was the devising of so-called stress rating scales, all of which explained stress as a reaction to making changes. Some of the assigned weights, or rankings of severity, assigned to various life experiences were intuitively anticipated; others were somewhat surprising. The highest-rated, most stress-creating events included major disruptions such as the death of a spouse or divorce.

Intermediate and moderately stressful rankings related to retirement, being fired from a job, a child's leaving home, and the start or end of formal schooling. Lower-ranking but still significant events involved changes in diet, recreation, social activities, and sleep. The significant factor, regardless of ranking, was that individuals were required to effect some kind of change in their lives.

These rating scales also approximated for statistical probability of the stressed individual's experiencing a health change within two years of a significant accumulation of life-change units. The higher an individual's stress "score," the higher the probability of a major health change, which could involve physical illness and/or psychological or psychiatric disorders.

At this point, you may be asking, "Why all the chatter about the stress on the caretaker when the brain-injured person is the one with the real problem?" Admittedly, the brain-injured person has suffered a catastrophic, life-altering experience, but is receiving appropriate intensive medical care and may not be lucid enough for many months to understand fully what has happened. The caregiver, on the other hand, must make critical decisions throughout the periods of hospitalization and rehabilitation, and then must provide constant, high-quality home care, with little or no prior experience. Unfortunately for the caregiver, all of this may transpire at a time of maximum vulnerability to stress-related deterioration of health. Further, if a high stress score is accumulated within a period of weeks or months, rather than years, then a health crisis can become all but inevitable.

Stress values run from 100 (death of a spouse) to 15 (changes in eating habits). In between are such events as the death of a close family member (63), change in the health of a family member (44), the beginning or end of school (26), and change of residence (20). Curiously, even changes that would normally be seen as positive figure on the stress scale; for example, marital reconciliation and outstanding personal achievement carry stress ratings of 47 and 28, respectively.

Though she was sometimes discouraged, Donna never despaired. Her faith and her support system helped her realize that the subconscious could be a strong ally in helping her to deal with potentially overwhelming events. She demonstrated an important principle that Selye recognized in his investigation of physiological responses: Given identical stresses, individuals' attitudes largely determined their physiological responses. One person might experience unbearable stress working eight hours at a job deemed boring and distasteful; another might thrive on working 12 hours a day at tasks deemed meaningful and rewarding. Ultimately, it was not the length of the workday or even the nature of the work that was significant; it was the worker's attitude that mattered.

Caregivers cannot reverse the past or its effects, but they can alter their response to them and thus can lessen the likelihood of a health crisis. As Donna altered her response to Eve's brain injury and the difficulty of helping her recover from it, she recognized the areas in which she had some control and those in which she had none. As she learned to live the Serenity Prayer, she began to function more effectively and became more creative in her management of Eve's rehabilitation.

Donna's intuitive grasp of the power of the subconscious made an enormous difference in the way she responded to her circumstances. Had she relied solely on the resources of her linear, logical conscious mind, she would soon have been overwhelmed, foundering at last in the useless and self-defeating entanglements of "what if." Enlisting the help of her subconscious mind enabled Donna to deal creatively with each new crisis in turn, and thus to preserve her serenity and sense of empowerment.

The psychologist Abraham Maslow proposed the following relationship between personal expectations and actual accomplishments:

$$\frac{\text{Accomplishments}}{\text{Expectations}} = \text{Self-Worth}$$

This model implies that if expectations are allowed to become greater than actual accomplishments, self-worth will suffer and be diminished; and once self-worth is diminished, the ability to accomplish will be further impaired. The only way to break this destructive cycle is by systematically lowering one's expectations. Our highly competitive, success-oriented culture would reject this stratagem, yet for all its astonishing simplicity, the stratagem works, and works well.

Drawing on her own life experiences and employing her hard-won wisdom in dealing with Eve, Donna made allowances for her limitations and, more important, for her ingenuity and considerable powers of will.

Recognizing the futility of unrealistic expectations, Donna all but eliminated the debilitating effects of stress. By acknowledging her ability to call forth and enlist the powers of hers and Eve's subconscious, she "improvised" a regimen that brought Eve back from helplessness to recovered strength and autonomy. Thus she accomplished what medical science implied she could not and proved that Eve's course was neither as fixed or destined as some would have had her believe.

# About the Authors

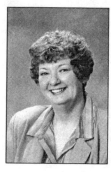

*Brain, Heal Thyself* is based on Madonna Siles's experience as the caregiver of her best friend, the survivor of a near-fatal brain aneurysm and strokes. Desperate to help her, Madonna developed a holistic rehabilitation plan, drawing on her experience as a practitioner of Λ.Λ.'s 12-Step program and her personal knowledge of subconscious communication techniques. She learned about the amazing power of the subconscious, and the various methods to invoke its help in the healing process, primarily from her friend and coauthor Lawrence J. Beuret, M.D. Last but not least, it is Madonna's belief that her 30-year career in the wild and wooly advertising business gave her the courage to combine creatively her knowledge and experience to form the "program" that helped save her friend from an invalid existence and her own sanity as a caregiver.

Madonna is a graduate of the University of Illinois, Champaign-

elor of science degree in communications. Visit
ativecaregiving.com.


; his private practice in 1973, Lawrence J. Beuret,
M.D., has helped hundreds of patients with psychosomatic (mind
and body) disorders to identify and alleviate the source of their
symptoms. Using a combination of medical and psychological therapies and subconscious communication techniques, Dr. Beuret works
with the patient to unravel the mysteries that cause many baffling
physical/psychological conditions: panic/anxiety, post-traumatic
stress and attention disorders, depression, anorexia symptoms, car-
diac neurosis, and irrational fears and phobias. His success has been
based on a drug-free, medically oriented approach to what is generally viewed to be a psychological condition.

Throughout his career, Dr. Beuret's work has attracted the attention of Chicago radio personalities and inspired coverage by the
local press. He has lectured and published medical journal articles
in both the United States and Europe on the lifelong effects of birth
trauma and methods of recalling unconscious early childhood memories. Currently, Dr. Beuret's practice is primarily devoted to drug-
free neurodevelopmental remediation for adults and children
suffering from attention and learning disorders.

Dr. Beuret is a graduate of Loyola University Stritch School of
Medicine in Chicago, and he received a fellowship in pediatrics for
his residency at the Mayo Clinic in Rochester, Minnesota. In addition, Dr. Beuret has continued his studies at the National Academy
of Medical Hypnosis in Atlanta, Georgia, and the Institute for Neuro-
Physiological Psychology in Chester, England.

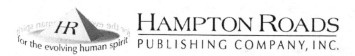

# HAMPTON ROADS
PUBLISHING COMPANY, INC.

Thank you for reading *Brain, Heal Thyself*. Hampton Roads is proud to publish an extensive array of books on the topics discussed in this book—topics such as health, caregiving, alternative therapies, and more. Please take a look at the following selection or visit us anytime on the web: www.hrpub.com.

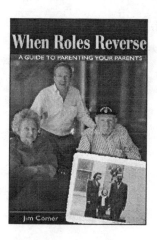

## When Roles Reverse
*A Guide to Parenting Your Parents*
Jim Comer

This is an indispensable guide for anyone in a caregiving situation. Comer shares the experiences of caring for both of his parents, while offering warmth, humor, and real-life advice designed to save you time, money, and tears.

Paperback • 288 pages
ISBN 1-57174-500-9 • $15.95

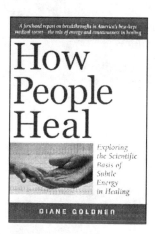

## How People Heal
*Exploring the Scientific Basis of Subtle Energy in Healing*
Diane Goldner

If you've ever gone to an energy healer or been curious about the process, this paperback reissue of Goldner's *Infinite Grace* is for you. Goldner goes in-depth with renowned healers, including Barbara Brennan and Rosalyn Bruyere, as well as the patients who use energy medicine to positive effect against everything from cancer to AIDS.

Paperback • 360 pages • ISBN 1-57174-363-4 • $14.95

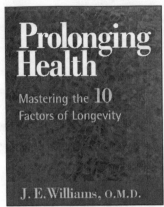

## Prolonging Health
### *Mastering the 10 Factors of Longevity*
J. E. Williams, O.M.D.

Based on the latest medical findings, Dr. Williams presents a practical, 10-point plan for anti-aging, using the best of natural medicine. He shows how to strengthen your heart, revitalize your brain, rebalance your hormones, repair your DNA, and more. This definitive guide includes important information on "Aging and the Brain," along with advice for having an informed talk with your doctor.

Paperback • 464 pages • ISBN 1-57174-338-3 • $17.95

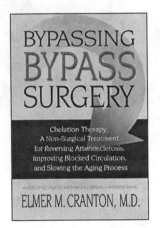

## *Bypassing Bypass Surgery*
Elmer Cranton, M.D.

This classic guide gives you the straight facts on chelation therapy, a safe alternative to bypass surgery that also offers benefits against stroke, circulatory problems, and more.

Paperback • 416 pages
ISBN 1-57174-297-2 • $17.95

# Hampton Roads Publishing Company

*. . . for the evolving human spirit*

HAMPTON ROADS PUBLISHING COMPANY publishes books on
a variety of subjects, including, spirituality, health,
and other related topics.

***For a copy of our latest trade catalog,***
call toll-free, 800-766-8009, or send your name and address to:

HAMPTON ROADS PUBLISHING COMPANY, INC.
1125 STONEY RIDGE ROAD • CHARLOTTESVILLE, VA 22902
e-mail: hrpc@hrpub.com • www.hrpub.com